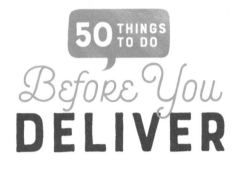

50 THINGS TO DO

Before You

DELIVER

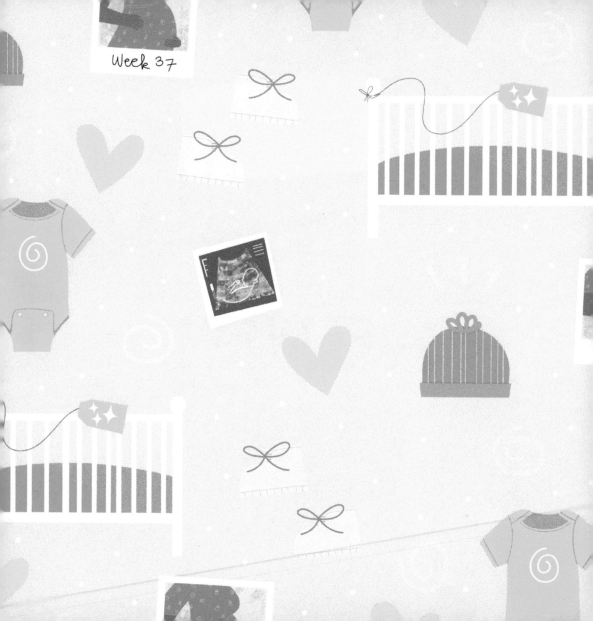

Week 37

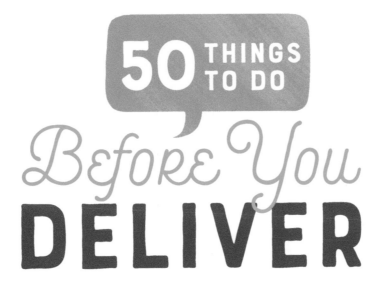

50 THINGS TO DO

Before You DELIVER

THE FIRST-TIME MOM'S PREGNANCY GUIDE

for Your Baby, Your Body, and Your Sanity

JILL KRAUSE

FOUNDER OF BABYRABIES.COM

Foreword by Sara A. Robert, MD

ROCKRIDGE
PRESS

For general information on our other products and services or to obtain technical support, please contact our Customer Care Department within the United States at (866) 744-2665, or outside the United States at (510) 253-0500.

Rockridge Press publishes its books in a variety of electronic and print formats. Some content that appears in print may not be available in electronic books, and vice versa.

Illustrations © 2018 by Alyssa Gonzalez

Author photo © Scott Krause

ISBN: Print 978-1-93975-410-3 | eBook 978-1-64152-097-3

*To every fellow parent
who has ever given me a knowing glance,
a gentle hug, or a kind comment
letting me know I'm not doing this alone.*

A B C

CONTENTS

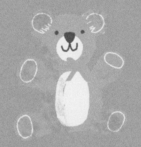

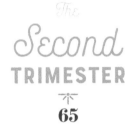
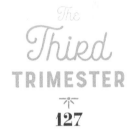

FOREWORD

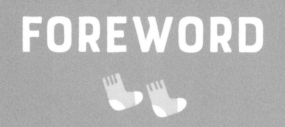

I have always told my patients that pregnancy is nine months for a reason. Some people think it gives you time to prepare your body and mind to become the perfect parent. Realistically, it's time to come to the realization that there's no such thing as a "perfect" parent. The nine-month period gives you a reasonable amount of time to come to accept, and maybe even embrace, imperfection. In those months, you will lose control of your time, your body, and (on some days) even your mind . . . a preview of what your new life as a mom will be.

An important aspect of my job is helping my patients get through both the most rewarding and worrisome time of their lives. I frequently make the joke that I should have board certifications in both OB-GYN *and* psychiatry. First-time moms-to-be are rightfully scared of the unknown: pregnancy, labor, delivery, breastfeeding, parenting, and so on. I often find myself talking patients off the ledge, so to speak, about something they read online or on a medical pregnancy app. This book makes my job easier. It gives women realistic expectations and guidance for some of these previously scary unknowns.

Although it sounds like a cliché, your goal in pregnancy should be "healthy mom, healthy baby." You can only do something about what you have control over, like eating a healthy diet and taking care of yourself. Look at the nine months of pregnancy as a test. What's important is not so much how well you score but how well you handle the loss of control.

When I was pregnant with my first child, I was a little "granola," but I was also a type A control freak who wanted to know what was going to happen 10 steps beforehand. One night when I was 39 and a half weeks along, I woke up around 11:00 pm. I felt like I needed to pee, so I got up and waddled to the bathroom. By the time I got there, the urge had gone away. I waddled back to the bed and, just when I was getting comfortable, the urge to pee returned. This back and forth went on for about an hour before I realized that it was happening every eight minutes. Only then did it occur to me that *this* was labor. I got in the shower, shaved my legs (of course), blow-dried my hair, and put on makeup. I woke up my husband and off we went to the hospital. Once we got to the labor and delivery floor, a nurse checked my cervix. Wide-eyed, she said, "Dr. Robert, you're dilated to seven centimeters!"—meaning, I was in active labor. I was a trained physician and everything was moving faster than I could process it. Any semblance of control I thought I had was gone. My baby was now in control . . . which was scary but also fantastic. That experience is still, to this day, one of the best of my life!

The patients I've seen who have the best pregnancy and labor experiences have been both well-prepared *and* open-minded. Jill's book is funny (as it's meant to be), but more importantly, it's reality. It's a guidebook to pregnancy that acts as a link between your healthcare provider, your family and friends' unsolicited advice, and all the crazy stuff you will read online. It's a useful tool that makes you laugh.

Because if you didn't laugh, you would probably be crying (those of you further into your pregnancy know what I'm talking about).

So work as a team with your medical provider, keep asking questions of your friends and family, and read as much as you can. Enjoy this book. Keep it on your bedside table or in your diaper bag. Pick it up when you need a pick-me-up. Use it to generate questions to ask your OB-GYN or midwife. The nine months of pregnancy are about preparing for the most challenging, rewarding, and amazing experience of your life. Don't let fear of the unknown take away from that.

SARA A. ROBERT, MD
Obstetrician and Gynecologist

INTRODUCTION

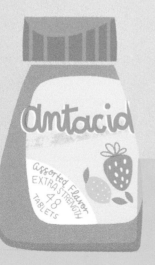

I called poison control on myself when I was eight weeks pregnant with my first baby. It was two o'clock in the morning.

Earlier that night, when I was getting ready for bed, I noticed an unopened bottle of Tums on our bathroom sink. It wasn't mine—it was my husband's. Before I was pregnant, I detested Tums. I'd sooner eat cat litter. But after an entire day of morning sickness and an inability to eat (or keep down) almost anything, those pastel tablets looked oddly appetizing.

My first instinct was to question my own judgment, and I did, ever so briefly. My second instinct—is there such a thing as a second instinct?—was to carry the bottle with me to bed, turn on a television show about someone else having a baby, and shove about 50 Tums into my mouth in 30 minutes. I did that, too. My third instinct is proof that we should always listen to the first instinct and go no further. I decided to see what the Internet had to say about eating 50 Tums in the amount of time it takes to watch someone else on TV push out a baby. This was a terrible idea. I went into panic mode after reading about all the diseases my baby and I were going to get, and that perhaps my baby would be born in a calcium shell. Enter poison control.

Luckily, a nice nurse on the other end of the line talked me down and assured me that the worst I could do was constipate myself. Phew! But, also, I learned that I really *shouldn't* make a habit of eating that many Tums in one sitting. Noted. Odds are, you too might have a second or third instinct wildly mislead you at some point soon. You are definitely not alone.

Confession time: I have been pregnant four times. Over the course of those four pregnancies, I've learned to balance a few things:

— The natural anxiety that comes with creating another human life
— The overwhelming alarmism parents get flooded with, especially when they go online
— Wisdom

It is a delicate balance. Nervousness is totally normal when you're pregnant.

This is a huge deal! It's easy to get bogged down and obsessed with search engine results when your mind is in overdrive trying to prepare for life with a baby. Resist the urge to get sucked in. Your body already knows what to do, and bodies have been doing this way longer than Google has been around. Instead, it's better to focus that nervous energy on practical tasks that will actually get you prepared to be, like, an adult who is in charge of a real live baby. You've got nine months to prepare, and I've got 50 things for you to get done.

Your Body, but Everybody's Baby

Over the course of your pregnancy, there will be no shortage of advice, both wanted and unsolicited, thrown at you. Grandparents, friends, pregnancy apps, your medical provider—they're all going to be telling you what you should and shouldn't be doing. And they probably all mean well, and most make excellent points, but it's totally okay to ignore Aunt Kay's advice to drink a bottle of castor oil at 39 weeks pregnant. In fact, it's fine for you to thank people for their advice with one breath and then laugh at them in your head the next (or maybe even out loud, because pregnancy rage is a thing).

It may take a village, but at the end of the day, this baby, this pregnancy, is yours.

The Info and Advice That Matter

Okay, you're probably wondering what makes me an authority on nailing down these 50 things for you. I'll remind you that nobody has the final say on what you should do while gestating, including me. This is not a blueprint for a perfect pregnancy. Perfection doesn't exist for parents, even in pregnancy. In fact, I'm fixated on setting the bar low and focusing on reality instead of perfection. Do you know why? *Because I have four kids!*

As I mentioned, I've been pregnant four times, and gave birth to my youngest baby a little over a year ago. On any given day, I'm arguing with a nine-year-old about why he can't play video games made for college kids, I'm begging my seven-year-old to please let me brush her ratty hair, I'm reminding my four-year-old to put his penis away when we're in public, and I'm breast-feeding a baby while he tries to pick my nose. The chaos is, inexplicably, part of the joy.

I've been blogging about pregnancy and parenthood for 10 years, since before I conceived my first baby. I bought the Internet domain name BabyRabies.com one night when I realized I actually had baby rabies. Baby rabies is like baby fever to the extreme—I was obsessed with getting pregnant. Over the course of a decade, I've evolved from a perfect parent—before I had my first child—to a real parent. Kind of like *The Velveteen Rabbit*, you know? I'm shabbier from all the love and life with my kiddos. My imperfections are impossible to hide. But in becoming a real parent, I realized I would never want to be a perfect parent now. It's better this way.

The goal of this book isn't to set you up to be a perfect parent or have a perfect pregnancy. The goal is to give you some actionable advice that will prepare you for real life with a baby and help you focus on taking care of YOU while you're pregnant and beyond.

I combined my 10 years of blogging, my talking online and offline with thousands of pregnant women and new moms, and my own experience with four pregnancies, and selected these 50 to-dos to focus on while your body handles the job of growing your baby. I specifically chose each one to help focus your anxious mind, to give your hands something to do, to give you things to look forward to (aside from that bundle of joy), to empower and uplift you, and to provide information you'll need to advocate for yourself for both your physical and mental health.

Don't stress about the timing of these things. While some tasks will coincide with specific weeks in your pregnancy, you should be able to work through most of this book at your own pace. If you're already well into your second trimester by the time you're reading this, you can still go back and work on tasks in the first trimester's to-dos. And if some things just sound like a terrible idea to you, I won't take it personally if you skip over them.

It's my hope that you will use this book to help you feel accomplished and in control as your pregnancy progresses, and that there will be several to-dos that never occurred to you and that wind up enriching your pregnancy experience in some way.

What to Expect When... Reading this Book

These tips, to-dos, and reminders cover a broad spectrum of what needs attention while you're pregnant. They're not just about creating a baby registry and fluffing your nest. There are tasks to help keep you healthy, to help you sleep, to ensure that you bond with your partner, to strengthen existing friendships, and to make new mom-friends. There are also some fun projects, maternity fashion tips, and photography tutorials throughout. This isn't meant to feel like a chore.

Are these to-dos everything you need to do while pregnant? No. There are some tasks, like deciding if you want genetic testing and searching for a childcare provider, that are going to be so specific to your individual circumstances that I can't really give you any useful insight. But I aim to help lighten your mental and emotional load through the to-dos that I am sharing so you can better focus on tasks that are deeply personal to you.

Some of my favorite parents and care providers have chimed in with their own tips, advice, and real-world words of wisdom. When I asked each of them to contribute, I told them I wanted them to tell me something they wish they had known when they were pregnant for the first time.

Some people in your circle are going to love to tell you that life as you know it is over, and everything is going to change, and, OMG, you will never be able to do what you want now that you're going to be a parent! It doesn't take a genius to know that babies change things, and you certainly don't need your cousin's unsolicited warnings to remind you. Instead of getting down about what you'll miss out on, this is a great time to check off some pregnancy bucket list adventures. There are some things you'll get to enjoy only while you're pregnant—like rocking that gorgeous belly bump in a bikini. And don't let the nine months pass by without documenting your pregnancy in some way. Your future self will thank you.

Pregnancy can be wondrous, pregnancy can be scary, pregnancy can be any human emotion you've ever felt. Whether you're reading this with joy in your heart, totally thrilled and ready to tackle the next nine-ish months, or you're overwhelmed and terrified about how you're going to make it through this, you are not alone. Just like there is no such thing as a perfect pregnancy, there is no right way to feel about it.

Take control of what you can, and roll with the rest. You've got this.

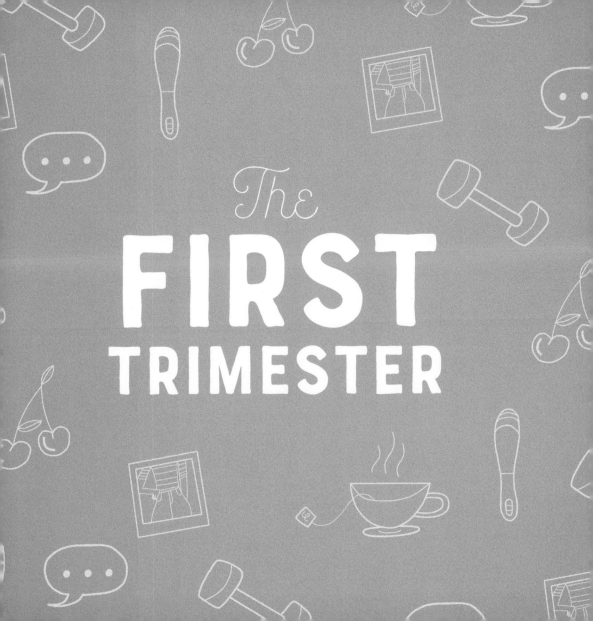

The
FIRST
TRIMESTER

It is the most
powerful creation
for you to be able to have life
growing inside of you.
There is no bigger gift,
nothing more empowering.

Beyoncé

When did you find out? Maybe you didn't realize you were pregnant for six weeks, eight weeks, or more. Or perhaps you're acutely aware of every minute that has passed since you ovulated. At a minimum, you are at least four weeks pregnant now. That's because the pregnancy clock starts on the day your cycle began, or the first day of your last period, not the day you conceived.

And that already feels like an accomplishment, right? It's like the first to-do was "Deal with your period like you've been doing since that awkward day in junior high," followed shortly by "Ovulate like a boss" and then "Make a baby." This book is all about helping you feel accomplished, so up top, lady—high five! You've already completed some pretty miraculous tasks. Check, check, check!

So now here you are, in your first trimester. This is the trimester when you feel super pregnant but don't really look pregnant. You may be exhausted, gassy, nauseous, and bloated. But you're probably not quite ready to tell the world that the reason you puked in your trash can and your pants don't fit isn't because you were the rock star who closed down the bar the night before and you've been eating too many nachos. It's business as usual on the outside and something along the lines of "Holy crap, my body is growing another person, and I think I'm going to pee my pants" on the inside.

Personally, I like this part. I mean, excessive peeing and toxic relationships with food aside, I like when people don't know I'm pregnant unless I tell them. It's a fun secret to keep from the rest of the world—while you still can.

Before we get any further, do you need a nap? Come on in, lay your cheek right here on this page. I got you, girl. Shhhhh, no one'll notice. In case nobody has told you this yet, it's totally normal to question how you're going to function, especially if you can't keep your eyes open now. Nap without shame whenever possible—the fatigue is legit, and while it may not look like you are doing much from the outside, you are on overdrive on the inside.

The first 14 to-dos in this trimester are all about laying the groundwork for a great pregnancy while also addressing the immediate changes happening to your body and your life. We'll cover the basics, like how to choose a medical provider for your pregnancy and delivery, and explore some morning sickness survival tips. We'll also get into the fun stuff, like how to announce your pregnancy and what baby gear to begin researching.

Remember, these are suggestions, and there's no failing Pregnancy 101 if you don't get through them over the next two months. Many of these can be accomplished later, in between naps.

As Queen Bey said at the beginning of this chapter, growing a baby can feel empowering, and I hope my guidance and support will help you feel empowered as you work through these to-dos. It's also okay and normal if you find this trimester less than magical at times. Stay true to who you are and what's important to you while your body does its thing.

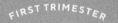

FIRST TRIMESTER

1

FIGURE OUT IF AN OB OR A MIDWIFE IS BEST FOR YOU

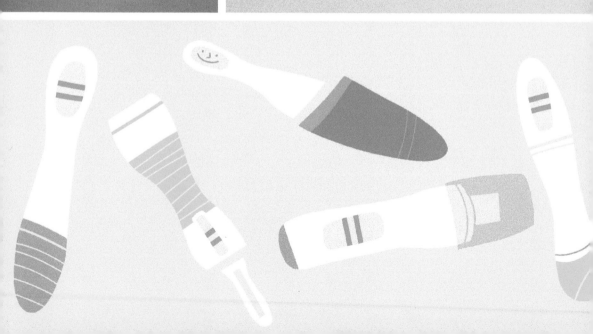

*T*he pee is dry on your pregnancy test— it's a yes—and now it's time to find a medical provider. This person will help you navigate your health and be there when you deliver your baby. Maybe you already know that you want to go with a traditional obstetrician-gynecologist (OB-GYN), or a midwife, or both. Maybe you've always wanted to deliver at home and so that's your goal right from the start. And maybe, just maybe, you have no clue where to start with the who, what, where, and why of these important decisions. Which is why we're beginning right here.

When I was four weeks pregnant with my first, I went to my primary care doctor, who confirmed the pregnancy by blood test, and then handed me a business card for an OB-GYN practice he recommended, and that was it! No pamphlets, no lists of things I shouldn't eat, nothing. I was a whole four weeks pregnant and didn't know what to do! Of course, there's really not much you *need* to do in those first four weeks, so you do have the time to research which professional you want to spend the next 36 weeks visiting frequently. This individual is going to have a big impact on how and where you give birth. Don't be like me and schedule an appointment with the obstetrician from the first business card you get. Had I researched that practice, I wouldn't have wasted 20 weeks (and way too many hours languishing in the waiting room past my appointment time) with that doctor.

When it comes to the pregnancy, no one wants to take chances. We all want a provider who is the absolute best, which is why it's really hard to accept the idea that choosing a health care provider isn't about which one is "the best." Some providers might have all the right professional degrees and still be wrong for you. What really matters is that you find a health care provider who is best for *you* and will work with *your* birth expectations. You have choices. OB-GYNs, certified nurse midwives (CNMs), and certified midwives (CMs) take care of women who choose to have an unmedicated/natural birth or a birth with pain medications or epidurals. So give some thought first to how and where, ideally, you want to bring your little one into the world, and consider provider options from there. Regardless of which type of provider you choose, ask questions and make an educated decision that's best for you.

UNDERSTANDING PROVIDERS

Jeanean Carter, certified nurse midwife

If you have what is considered a "high-risk" pregnancy (for example, multiple gestation or insulin-dependent diabetes), then the safest place for delivery is a hospital setting. In this case, an obstetrician or a CNM or CM who works with an OB would be the best choice. If a cesarean delivery is needed, a physician is required.

For low-risk pregnancies, there are options when choosing a health care provider and birth location. Midwives or labor and delivery nurses can provide labor and birth support regardless of whether or not the labor is medicated. Midwives are skilled and experienced in helping women with a variety of birthing positions, including standing, squatting, or on the hands and knees. They also have experience in water birth deliveries, whether it be in a tub or the shower. Most physicians do not have experience with water births or out-of-bed births. If birthing in a non-hospital setting, in alternative positions, or if water is important to you, a midwife may be the best fit.

THE RIGHT PROVIDER

Jen McLellan, founder of PlusSizeBirth.com

If you're a plus-size mom, connecting with a size-friendly care provider can make a big impact on the care you receive. You can ask your provider questions like "What has been your experience working with women of size?" Or "Will you classify me as high risk based only upon my weight?" (Hint: The answer here should be no!)

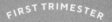

FIRST TRIMESTER

2

PREPARE TO COMBAT MORNING SICKNESS

Chamomile

*W*hile some lucky pregnant women manage to escape any kind of morning sickness, many of us will feel it to some degree. And it doesn't always show up in the morning. Of course, sometimes, just like in the movies, morning sickness symptoms are the very reason we discover we're harboring an embryo.

In fact, mine tended to last all day and would get worse in the evening. Not everyone throws up. Some people feel waves of nausea, or they might feel like they're on the verge of throwing up nearly all the time. If you're still very early in your pregnancy, any nausea that occurs probably won't set in until a few weeks after your positive pregnancy test.

As for the remedies, a lot of moms-to-be seem to have one special morning sickness trick that works for them, but since all our experiences are totally unique, it's impossible to know exactly which trick will work for you. Welcome to this confusing thing called pregnancy!

Planning ahead will help prepare you if and when you get morning sickness, or afternoon sickness, or evening sickness, or all-day sickness. It's no fun to wait until you are in the thick of it to try and figure out what will help you feel better. Many moms find that an empty stomach makes them feel sick, so try to keep bland snacks on hand at all times, including when you're out of the house. Foods that fall into the general categories of sour, tart, salty, bland, cheesy, spicy, and bubbly can help with morning sickness. Pop some in your purse; keep a stash on your nightstand so you can get something in your stomach before you even get out of bed.

MEDICAL TIP

There's a difference between typical pregnancy sickness and its more extreme form, called hyperemesis gravidarum (HG). HG is a less common malady, but one that could require medical intervention and intravenous fluid hydration. If you're experiencing severe and frequent vomiting and food aversions, notify your medical provider. For more information, check out Hyperemesis.org.

Here's a shopping list so you can stock up now on some items that have been known to help expectant moms (or if it's too late, give this list to your support person to shop for you while you take a nap by your toilet). This list covers it all—try out these options and stick with what works for you.

- Bread for toast
- Chamomile tea
- Cinnamon disc candy, cinnamon gum
- Fizzy fruit sodas
- Ginger chews, ginger candy, ginger ale
- Graham crackers
- Lemon drop candies
- Lots of fresh lemons for lemon water
- Macaroni and cheese
- Mashed potatoes (the instant kind do the trick for me), plus grated cheese to melt over them
- Olives
- Peppermint candy, peppermint tea
- Pickles
- Saltine crackers
- Sour Patch Kids candies
- Sparkling water
- Vitamin B_6 (ask your health care provider first)

If morning sickness equals puke for you, but you're expected to leave the house and be presentable, here are some preventative measures you can take:

In your car. Keep a towel within reach and a bucket nearby in case you need to hurl mid-gridlock. Also, pack a spare outfit in a plastic bag in case you need to change. Yes, a whole outfit, including clean undies; the force of throwing up might make you pee.

In your purse. Pack a spare toothbrush and toothpaste, some breath mints, lip balm, face-cleansing wipes, and, if needed, a hair tie.

WATER
YOUR NEW BEST FRIEND

It's important to stay hydrated throughout pregnancy, especially if you're having a hard time keeping food down right now. Do you have a water bottle or insulated cup that you love yet? If not, treat yourself to one, and commit to being BFFs with it. It should be easy to clean, keep your water cold (unless you don't like cold water), fit in your bag and car cup holder if you travel frequently, and be easy to hold and drink from with one hand. Not only will a great water bottle or cup serve you well through pregnancy, but it will also get you through life with a sleeping newborn in one arm and only one hand free to quench your thirst. And if you end up breastfeeding? Words can't even describe how thirsty you're going to be—your kid will literally be siphoning the fluid from your body. My personal favorite is a stainless steel, double-wall 20-ounce cup with a watertight lid that also accommodates a straw. It's easier to drink from a straw without waking a sleeping baby, or spilling on them.

3

DOWNLOAD PREGNANCY APPS

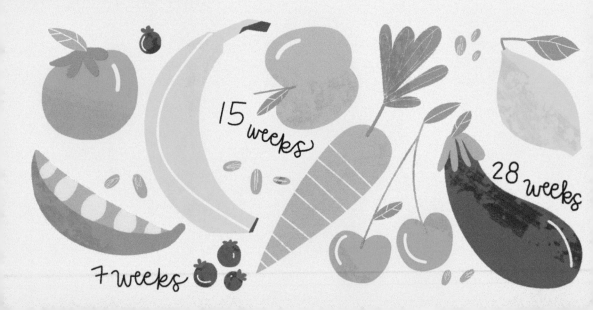

15 weeks

28 weeks

7 weeks

*W*hether it's for gestating, naming, or birthing a baby, there is literally an app for that part of the process. Take advantage of technology and download some apps that will help you keep track of and document the next nine-ish months.

There are four main categories of pregnancy apps: baby growth trackers, pregnancy photo apps, baby-naming apps, and contraction and delivery apps—and many options within each. Here is what I think makes for a good app in each of these categories, and you can pick what works best for you and whatever technology you're rocking.

Baby growth tracker apps

You can get so much out of a baby growth tracker app. Full of fun features, like telling you what size veggie or pastry your baby is that week, these clever apps can help you calculate an estimated due date even before you've had your first prenatal appointment. Many also give you a weekly play-by-play of how and what your baby is developing that week (like fingers and toes), what you should be feeling and experiencing, and some things to look out for or questions to ask your medical provider.

Look for apps that are fun and make you smile, but also be sure they are created by reputable websites or brands. They shouldn't ever be a replacement for medical advice, but you should be able to trust what you're reading. Also, if an app makes you feel panicked with too much or alarming information, ditch it. There are plenty of others to choose from, and simple may be better in this case.

Pregnancy photo apps

These help you keep track of that growing bump by reminding you to take belly pictures weekly or monthly using the camera on your phone. Some allow you to send your pictures privately to friends and family via e-mail. Most allow you to share them to your social media platforms.

Most photo apps give you the option to overlay words and art on each photo to commemorate moments like "Baby's first kick!" So if that's your thing, find one with graphics you like. Also, many of these will continue to serve you after baby is born, so check out what options they have for moments like "Baby's first smile."

Baby-naming apps

I find that people either love or hate picking out baby names. It can be super fun or polarizing and difficult. Like all things related to your pregnancy, people have opinions and are gonna share them. Decide whether you want to let them in on your thoughts or take their advice on naming.

Gone are the days of having to thumb through and highlight baby names in a book—though you still can do that, too. There are many baby-naming apps, so I'd look for one that lets you link accounts with your partner so you can compare which names your partner likes (and doesn't), and one that generates new names based on names you already like.

Contraction-timing and fetal-kick-counter apps

You're not going to need these for several months, but they are fun to start checking out. Of course, you won't use the contraction timer until you're nearing your delivery date. But in the meantime, many contraction-timing apps also offer fetal-kick-counting features. You'll get more use out of these. It's recommended that you start keeping track of fetal kicks around the end of your second trimester.

Ease of use is important here. For contraction timing, it helps to have a giant button that you have to push only at the beginning and then again at the end of each contraction. Check out the reporting features each app offers, too. If you're into graphs and line charts, you're in luck—there are lots of fun reports to geek out over.

This is just the beginning of what's out there in app-land for pregnant parents. There are prenatal exercise apps, water intake tracker apps, and more being introduced all the time. In fact, searching for pregnancy apps was one method I used to take my mind off first-trimester nausea. In the interest of not dating this book, I've avoided listing specific apps, but visit BabyRabies.com/PregnancyApps to find my absolute favorites, which I'm continually updating.

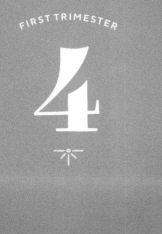

FIRST TRIMESTER

4

START TAKING CARE OF THE GODDESS YOU ARE

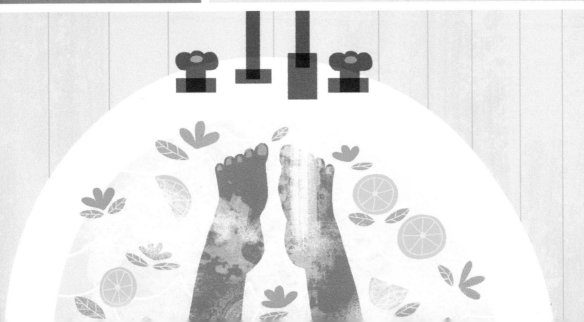

*H*ey, mama. How are YOU doing right now? Are you feeling a little overwhelmed or anxious, or maybe both? Maybe you're not allowing yourself to feel anything because you're so focused on keeping that little baby safe and sound? That's all totally normal. Let's chat about how you can start making space for you—a whole and separate person— while still taking care of that tiny person growing inside of you.

Your eight week appointment is going to be a big one. You'll likely have an ultrasound, a Pap smear, and many vials of blood taken. There are other tests and screenings you may opt for in this trimester, as well. Even if you don't get sweaty and queasy at the thought of needles in your arm, all this can be a lot to take on.

On that note, this is a great time to start arming yourself with some self-care techniques and keeping up old ones that will see you through your motherhood journey. These might include massages, meditation or breathing exercises, warm foot soaks, and a relaxing bedtime ritual.

I liked to give myself something fun to focus on after each appointment, so I used appointment days as "me" days. I took myself out to lunch for whatever I was craving at the moment, which was especially rewarding on the days they took blood for labs.

Some people like appointments to learn more about what's going on and get answers to their growing list of questions; others don't enjoy the waiting or the poking and prodding. Regardless, you can make appointment days something special:

- Bring a new magazine or book to your appointment.
- Bring a journal or a coloring book to work on while you wait.
- Schedule a post-appointment mani-pedi or haircut.
- Treat yourself to coffee or a snack at your local bakery on your way home or back to the office.

When your loved ones are excited to celebrate news of the baby and ask if you need anything, don't be afraid to ask for specific things, like those magazines or coloring books, for you! Or simply ask them to be there for you on days you need someone to talk to or even to attend appointments with.

THE BEST FRIEND TRICK

Greame Seabrook, certified life coach for moms

Whenever you get scared, anxious, or you start to judge yourself, stop and use the best-friend trick. Ask yourself this question:

"If my best friend were feeling like this, what would I do or say to help?"

This is a time to be gentle with yourself, mama. Remember that there is no right way to do pregnancy. Focus on you. It may seem like the minute you tell anyone you're pregnant you disappear, and all they see is a belly and a baby. You're still there. You're still important. Not because of the baby; because you are YOU. Cover the basics—eat well, stay hydrated, get rest. But also add in some fun. There's no reason you can't watch cat videos on YouTube while getting blood drawn, or get into a GIF war on Facebook while waiting for your doctor. You are allowed to still be silly or intense, happy or determined, quiet or the life of the party. You are still you.

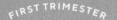

5

SHAKE OFF
ANY THOUGHTS
OF FIRST-TRIMESTER FRUMP

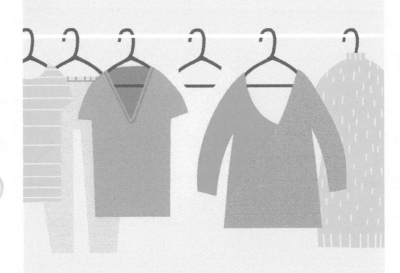

*A*s your hormones start taking control, you might start feeling pretty blah about your body. Perhaps you're not glowing, not showing, and you haven't broken out this bad since you were in high school. To you, the bloat is real, and the frump is here. Time to shake it off, hold your head up, and feel and look like the goddess you are.

Friend, it is even time to embrace elastic-waist pants. If your body is doing exactly what it's supposed to be doing—growing—do not keep trying to stuff yourself into your prepregnancy skinny jeans. You can do the rubber band around the button and through the buttonhole trick for a bit. But honestly? Get yourself some stretchy pants.

"But, Jill," you're saying, "I don't fit into maternity pants yet!" Right, I know. So buy (or borrow) transition pieces. They will transition you from your regular clothes *into* maternity clothes and then, after you've had your baby, they'll transition you *out of* your maternity clothes, making them great fourth-trimester clothes. (Note: That final transition can take as long as you need.)

What's a transition piece? Anything with a stretchy waist, a size larger than you normally wear, is a great place to start. Your boobs are probably inflating by the minute now, too, so sizing up in shirts is also a good idea. Something to keep in mind is whether those tops will be breastfeeding friendly if you plan to breastfeed your baby. Tops with deep V-necks, cross-front tops, or anything you can unbutton or easily pull down are all great fourth-trimester options. Choosing pieces that work now as well as then means you get double duty out of them.

Many women find that their skin breaks out terribly in the first trimester. Thanks a lot, hormones! Go easy on yourself, go makeup-free whenever you can, and keep your face clean—if you're too tired for a makeup removal ritual, keep facial cleansing wipes by your bed. Conversely, if you're feeling extra energetic, try making a simple oatmeal mask with equal parts of plain Greek yogurt, honey, and uncooked oats. Rub the mask on your face, let set for 10 to 15 minutes, then gently rinse.

While you may opt to go makeup-free at this point, don't skip the SPF. Your pregnant skin is actually more susceptible to the sun's rays and prone to discoloration known as melasma or "pregnancy mask." It can darken the skin on your forehead, cheeks, and upper lip, and usually takes a few months to fade after you've had your baby.

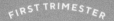

FIRST TRIMESTER

6

GET TALKING WITH YOUR PARTNER

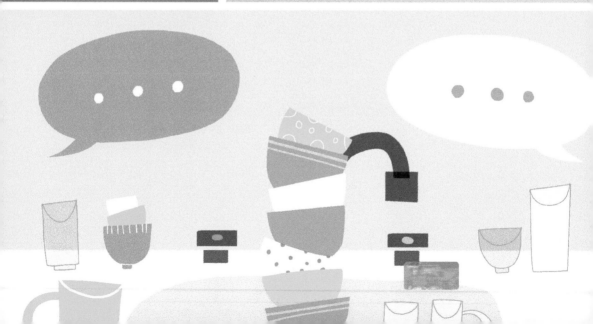

*I*f you are coupled, the key to making it through pregnancy and parenthood together is communication, and there's no time like the present.

Conversations with your partner right now may be mostly musings about what color eyes your baby will have and what totally random food you're hard-core craving, but there's a lot more to open up to each other about that will help you be a more successful team.

Coordination of prenatal appointments

Now is a great time to determine which appointments you'd like your partner to be there for, and which ones they can't make. Look ahead at their work calendar to see if any conflicts fall around the 18th to 20th week of your pregnancy. This is when your big ultrasound will be scheduled—you can see the baby really well and find out the gender if you want—so it's probably the one appointment you most want them to attend with you.

One of you might be thinking that both of you should be at every appointment and the other could be thinking that's not feasible. Don't assume that because you'll be raising a child together that you can read each other's minds. Talk it out.

Division of labor—before labor

Chances are you're prying your eyeballs open just to read this right now (so thank you, and I'm sorry). "Exhausted" doesn't even cover how tired some women feel in the first trimester. It's completely normal to give up on caring about things like clean laundry, washed dishes, and basic hygiene in favor of sleep. Be sure your partner understands that this is a normal reaction to growing an entire other human, and talk about some ways they can help with your share of the household duties while you're busy creating a life. Or just get on the same page about living in a dump for a while, and stock up on paper plates next time you're out.

S-E-X

If there's one thing you can count on during pregnancy, it's that you can't count on feeling the same one day to the next. This especially applies to sex. The combination of hormones, exhaustion, emotions, and your expanding belly and other parts of your body all make it impossible to predict when you'll want to make bedroom eyes versus murderous eyes at your partner when they try to hold your hand.

Plenty of women say their sex drive ramps up during pregnancy, and if that's you, AMAZING. Enjoy! But it's also common to feel exactly the opposite. Make sure your partner knows that both ends of the spectrum should be expected, even on a daily basis, and that it's not personal.

7

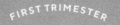

FIND
YOUR
VILLAGE

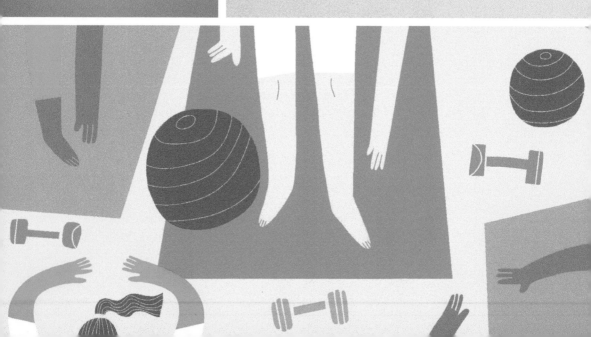

*F*rom the very beginning of your pregnancy, you may find a lot of comfort in knowing you're not alone when it comes to stuff you never knew would happen while incubating your future tax write-off. If you don't have other women you can confide in and ask if it's normal for your nipples to get THAT big, pregnancy can feel a bit isolating, especially if you're the first of your siblings, or the first person in your social circle, to experience it.

For as much as the media likes to perpetuate the "mommy wars," I have to say that, in my experience, most moms just want to find others they can relate to. We want to hear "Me too!" when we post on Facebook that we love our newborn baby so much but that we also really miss happy hour and regular showers. If you don't have a group of close IRL (in real life) family and friends who are already parents or are currently pregnant, you can try to make friends with some:

Stalk pregnant women in the pickle aisle. It's cliché, I know, but that's because it's SO TRUE. Hopefully, they'll notice your belly, which may just be bloat and leggings at this point, but roll with it. While not the most practical way to make new friends, this technique will come in handy in a few years when you develop a mom crush on the put-together-but-still-looks-like-she-struggles-with-mornings-too gal at the park with the only other three-year-old.

Sign up for a prenatal exercise class. Despite the fact that you'll have to exercise, this is an easy way to immerse yourself in an environment where at least you're guaranteed to meet other women in your area who are pregnant. You're also all bound to embarrass yourselves at some point if you go to classes together long enough, and nothing helps bond people in friendship like uncontrollable farting while stretching and accidentally peeing your yoga pants in front of each other.

Join a pregnancy message board or find moms on social media. There are pros and cons to seeking out an online village. It's easy to find others who are due around the same time as you are, and this is a fun outlet during pregnancy and beyond. I made a lot of online friends when I was pregnant with my first. We were all due around the same time, within about six months of each other. Nine years later, I'm still friends with many of them, and it's amazing watching all our kids grow up alongside each other online. That said, it is the Internet, and it can be a breeding ground for drama. Set boundaries, and don't get caught up in gossip or mean girl stuff. There are plenty of mature, intelligent adults to be found online. You may not be able to get together with your online friends for playdates at each other's houses after your babies are born, but you all clearly know how to use the Internet, and you'll be able to stay in touch for years to come.

Use social media to find local moms. For the best of both the online and offline worlds, seek out Facebook groups and apps that match you with other local moms whom you can meet up with offline for coffee now, and have newborn playdates with in your PJs in nine months.

You could also find you already have built-in parent friends throughout your family tree. Pregnancy can pave the way for deeper connections with family members, and you may find that your second cousin or your older sister becomes your new best mom-friend.

CONNECT LOCALLY

from Kacia Hosmer, blogger at Coconut Robot

I love how social media, like Instagram, can bring you together with like-minded people in motherhood when you are perhaps surrounded by those who aren't, but I am intentional about also finding people who are local, and I encourage my Instagram friends to do the same. You can't rearrange your messy house so that they only see a clean corner when they come over for coffee, and that realness is an important piece of friendships and connection with other moms.

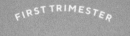

8

BEGIN A BABY NAMES LIST

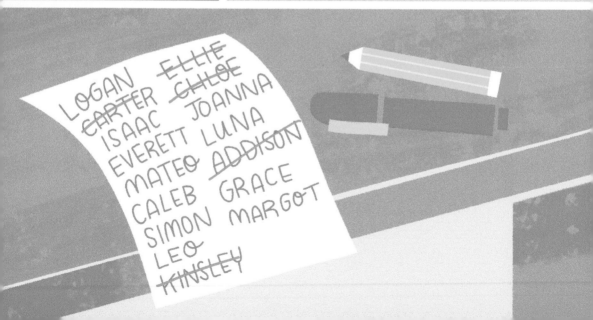

*W*hen I was 16, I thought I knew for sure what I would name my two perfect future children. I practiced writing their names in the margins of my school notes. By the time I needed to actually name a real baby 11 years later, those names were not even on the list of considerations. In fact, my list was basically blank. Naming a baby can be HARD when the baby isn't imaginary and you've lived long enough for other people and pop culture to ruin your once-favorite names.

Now, I know some of you are totally naming this baby that perfect name you dreamed up when you were in high school. Or maybe you've always had a family name in mind. I'm envious of you! Feel free to skip this section and enjoy this part of pregnancy being stress-free.

But if you're sticking around because you are totally at a loss and have no idea where to start when it comes to giving a little person a name that will represent who they are for the rest of their lives, deep breath. We're going to work through this.

As mentioned earlier, there are some great baby-naming apps on the market. Some even make it easy to connect accounts with your partner so you can collaborate on creating lists. Definitely take advantage of technology here!

But one of my favorite ideas for working together on a list of names is so low-tech that all you need is a bathroom mirror and a dry-erase marker or two. It goes like this:

- Write a name you like on the mirror anytime it strikes you. Your partner can wipe the name off if they don't like it. They can add their own favorites, and you can wipe those off.

- If you are super in love with a name, put a star next to it. If you put a star next to it, nobody can wipe it off without having a conversation about it.

- If you're not sure what the sex of the baby is, you can use different-color markers for boy names and girl names.

I love this because it's simple, it's fun, it's easy to update, and it's in a central location that you both have access to. I also love the idea of taking pictures of this list as it evolves. This strategy works if you're naming the baby on your own, too.

But baby names don't have to come from a book character, a family member, or an app. Here are some other sources of inspiration:

TV show or movie credits. This is how we named one of our four kids. When I was about 14 weeks pregnant with my third baby, I saw the name Lowell pop up in the credits of *Parenthood*, one of my all-time favorite shows. I loved it so much from the second I noticed it that I was scared to suggest it to my husband. Luckily, he immediately and enthusiastically said yes to it! From that moment, I was convinced I was going to have a girl because it was way too easy to pick out a boy's name.

Names of authors. Grab a coffee, head to a local bookstore, and make it a date.

Headstones in cemeteries. Yes, really—old names are making a comeback! Maybe stop by a local cemetery on your way home from the bookstore to finish off what will probably be one of the most unique dates you've ever been on.

Extended family trees. This is especially fun if anyone in your family is working on genealogy. You may love your great-great-great-uncle's name!

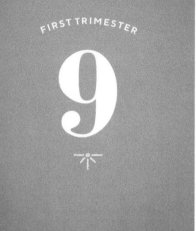

FIRST TRIMESTER

9

GEEK OUT OVER

BABY STUFF

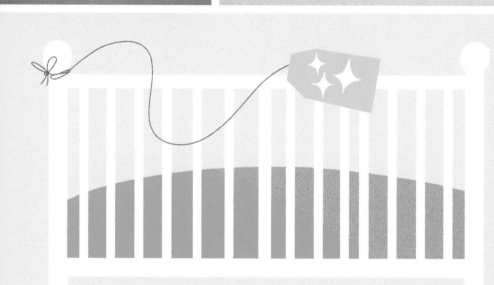

*O*ne of the most exciting parts of pregnancy is dreaming up how you'll decorate the baby's space and envisioning what stroller you'll push them in. It might be a little early to buy much of this, but it's not too early to learn more and get totally excited about it.

Head to a nearby baby store, or go on the Internet, and prepare to be amazed. If you haven't immersed yourself in the world of baby gear up until now, I bet you'll be shocked at all the things that claim to make life with baby easier. Before you get overwhelmed, remember that the majority of this stuff is not a necessity, and you'll have plenty of time to research what will work best for you. What follows is a handful of considerations.

Sleeping

Will your baby have a room of their own, or will they be rooming with you? Considering that space, would a full-size crib or a mini-crib make more sense? If the baby will sleep in another room, do you need an additional co-sleeper or portable crib for your room or for visiting the grandparents? These come in especially handy for road trips, as well as for those first few months when you'll probably be dealing with frequent night feedings.

Transporting

What kind of stroller will work best for your lifestyle, or do you even need one? If you live in the city and take public transportation a lot, you may want to opt to babywear most of the time—that is, wear baby in a sling or carrier—or you might get a stroller that is lightweight and folds easily if you'll be going up and down stairs often. If you live in the suburbs and will be loading a stroller in and out of the trunk of your vehicle, you'll need an option that fits in your car.

Diapering

How do you plan to diaper your baby? If you are considering cloth diapers, now is a great time to start researching what style of cloth diaper will work best for you, and calculating how much a full stash will cost. Even if you don't plan to cloth diaper full time, having a small stash on hand can be helpful for emergencies, like when you discover suddenly that you don't actually have another pack of diapers in the drawer at 2:00 a.m. Also, sometimes babies have allergic reactions to disposable diapers, and it's good to have cloth to transition them to while you try to figure out which brand of disposables will be best for them. In terms of cloth diapers, these are your options:

Flat and prefold diapers, paired with covers. These are the cloth diapers our parents remember. The difference is that we don't use giant diaper pins to close them anymore; instead, we place them in covers that close with Velcro® or snaps. A low-cost way to try out cloth diapering, they can be sized to fit nearly any baby. They don't go on as quickly as some other options, but they're easy to figure out

Fitted diapers, paired with covers. These can be more absorbent and don't require any kind of special folding. One size usually doesn't fit all, though, and they are more expensive than flats.

Pocket diapers. Once the pocket is stuffed with an insert, pocket cloth diapers go on and come off much like disposable diapers. Stuffing the diapers is an additional step, but the inserts allow you to adjust the diaper's absorbency, making them great for nighttime.

All-in-one diapers. These are usually the most expensive option, but they're also the easiest to use. There is nothing to stuff, and no additional cover needed. It's just what it says it is—all-in-one.

If you like the idea of cloth diapers and don't have the time or ability to commit to diaper laundry, but do have the financial resources, consider a local diaper service. They will drop off clean diapers, and launder your dirty diapers, usually weekly. They provide the diapers for you, so if this is something you think you'll end up using, don't stress about buying diapers for yourself.

THE CLUTCH CLOTH

Katie Barrington, mom of two

I love using cloth for the simple fact that they're always there. I don't have to run to the store in the rain or in the middle of the night when I'm elbow deep in breast milk poop. And I don't feel like I'm literally throwing money in the garbage can when my baby poops two seconds after I change her.

10

START DOCUMENTING

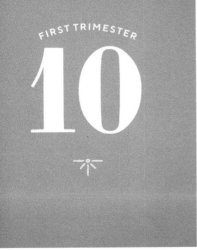

week 5

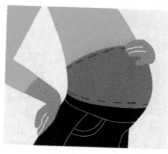

week 24

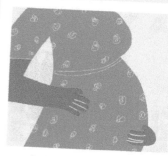

Week 37

*P*regnancy is a time of great change, and I'm not just talking about your growing belly and shockingly dark nipples. You're probably experiencing lots of feels these days. Maybe you're craving an outlet to write them down and work through, or maybe you just want to journal the experience.

You can go high tech, old school, or both, but consider documenting your pregnancy beginning as early as possible, even if you never intend for anyone to see or read it other than yourself and maybe your child, years from now. This time is fleeting, and you'll never get these thoughts, feelings, and this belly bump silhouette back.

Weekly or monthly belly pictures

It takes desire, a bit of commitment, and some follow-through, but taking a picture of your growing belly each week or each month can give you something to look forward to now, and a beautiful visual to look back on in the future. For the best continuity, try to take the photos in the same lighting, in the same spot, and in the same side-profile pose each time. Some moms are able to take them in the same outfit each time, too, by starting off wearing a super-stretchy top and pants. After baby is born, you can take one more picture, holding the newborn in front of your tummy where they once took up space on the inside. Then pop all the photos into iMovie or a time-lapse app in order, and watch your belly grow!

Note: Belly pictures do not have to be taken weekly, monthly, in the same outfit, or in the same spot to become future treasures. Just try to take pictures. You might very well hate them right now, but don't delete them! You'll cherish them one day. I promise.

An Instagram account

So maybe you're hip to the Insta already, and your followers fully expect you to totally document your pregnancy and beyond for all of them to see. Awesome. If not, or if you don't feel all that comfortable sharing with the rando who followed you after that time you met at a tailgate party, I offer this suggestion: Start a new Instagram account with the sole purpose of journaling and sharing this pregnancy (and this baby) to your heart's content. You can make it private. Heck, you don't even have to tell people about it! It's a great place to upload those belly pictures, with useful photo editing tools and filters to boot, and you can continue to share photos and thoughts of other moments along the way. But don't stop there. Get those pictures and thoughts into print. Many services allow you to link to your Instagram account and easily and inexpensively print photo books, prints, and even canvases.

An old-fashioned diary

The beauty of writing down your thoughts, fears, feelings, and letters to your unborn baby in a simple paper journal is that it's personalized, it won't get lost in a digital cloud, you don't need a password to access it or protect it, and you can put it in your baby's memory box (see page 79) for them to read when they get older.

No matter how you choose to document your pregnancy, I encourage you to be honest and honor the lows along with the highs. It's okay to write about what really scares you. It's okay to take pictures of the days you're feeling miserable. It's okay to document your cankles and the fight you and your partner got into over what baby name to choose. You're creating a life, not a Hallmark movie.

HASHTAGGING

If you think there is even a small possibility that this baby will have a sibling someday, don't name the Instagram account anything specific to just this baby. Instead, come up with a baby-specific hashtag; for example, baby's first and middle name if it's not a super-common combo (#WallaceAustin), or you can incorporate baby's nickname, like #PepperGrows. Just check if that hashtag is already being used!

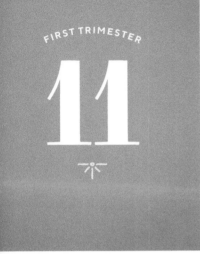

FIRST TRIMESTER

11

ANNOUNCE YOUR PREGNANCY

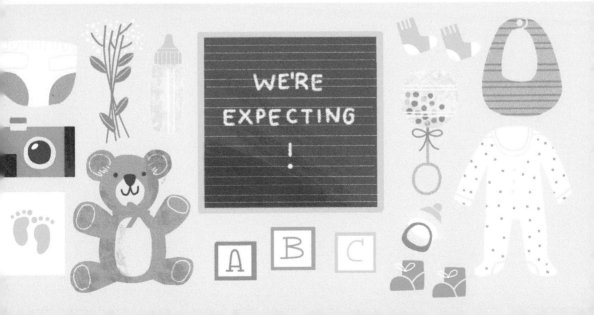

*T*he timing of the big reveal is very personal. Some people like to announce their pregnancy as soon as the pee dries on the pregnancy test, and some wait until they can't possibly hide it anymore. Between those two ends of the spectrum, many choose to announce their pregnancy toward the end of the first trimester or the beginning of the second trimester, once they've had one or two ultrasounds.

No matter what time feels more comfortable to you to let the world in on your huge secret, there are fun and cute ways you can make the announcement. A simple search for "pregnancy announcement" on Pinterest will take you to what seems like endless options and ideas. Keep in mind that no matter how you choose to tell the world, your inner circle will definitely appreciate hearing it from you in person rather than seeing it on social media (more on that later). That said, here are a few of my favorites:

The flat lay photo. Spell out all the details on a letter board or with chalk on a blackboard, arrange cute baby things around it, and take a photo from directly above. Send the photo by text and e-mail, and post it on social media.

The hidden-message photo. Take a photo of your favorite spot in the house with a pacifier in the foreground, or a picture of your dog bringing you a tiny pair of shoes. Say nothing else when you share it, and see how long it takes people to pick up on its real meaning.

The family videoconference call. This is especially great when you have family spread out all over the place. Use a group videoconferencing service to get everyone on your computer screen at once. Then none of them can be upset that they found out after someone else. Plus, you'll have the option of recording their reactions.

The personal gift. Tell baby's grandparents by gifting them a box of small baby items—think pacifiers, blankets, small toys—to keep at their house for future visits.

The telling tee. Casually walk into a family dinner rocking a "Does this shirt make me look pregnant?" tee, or something equally telling. No need to figure out what to say. Let the shirt do the work for you, and be sure your partner is ready with the camera to get video and photos of people's reactions.

If grand gestures really aren't your thing, that's fine, too. A pregnancy announcement doesn't count any less if you simply call people up and tell them the good news. I encourage you to share the news in person or over the phone first with close family and friends before sharing social media announcements with the world. This seems to matter a lot, especially to the older generation, who aren't so down with the idea of getting major announcements from those they love via their newsfeed.

WHEN THEY GO LOW

Jessica Martin-Webber, creator of The Leaky Boob *blog*

When people respond negatively to our pregnancy announcements, I tell them, "When you react like that, I don't want to include you in the happy news in my life because I feel hurt and like I can't trust you with my happy news. I didn't ask for your approval, but I do ask for your kindness and respect."

12

ASK FOR GOOD ADVICE

AND DODGE UNSOLICITED ADVICE

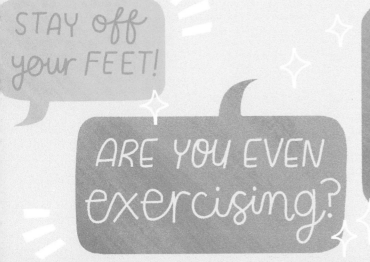

"Oh, honey, you need to stay off your feet." "Are you exercising? You don't want to put on too much weight!" "Wow! Your belly looks really small. Are you eating enough?"

Sigh. Just another day in the life of a pregnant woman. Once you start gestating, it's like your body and baby becomes everyone else's business. A lot of the advice that will be thrown at you, solicited or not, is well-meaning, but so much of it is also coming from a place of personal bias and not always backed by facts and science.

But, certainly, pregnancy can be confusing, and you can glean only so much knowledge from books (sorry, I'm trying!). How do you separate the good advice from the bad—and keep a sense of humor doing it?

Ask specific people for specific advice. Your best friend who breastfed three kids is an awesome resource to ask about breastfeeding, but she's not going to be the best person to turn to with questions about maternity leave if she hasn't worked outside of the home in 12 years.

Ask for and consider opposing points of view. You may be convinced that you want to cloth diaper 100 percent of the time, but it's also helpful to listen to friends who opted to use disposable diapers and find out what kept them from considering cloth diapers. This way, if someone says, "Have you considered that this won't work?" you're prepared to respond that, yes, you actually have.

Value the advice of medical professionals. Unless your great-aunt or your neighbor is an OB or a midwife, your actual OB or midwife is a better resource, because they are current on medical recommendations and standards of care. Write your questions or concerns down or keep them in a notes app on your phone, and spend part of each appointment taking advantage of your time with them to talk through your questions.

You do you. You may have to practice and focus on this skill early and often in motherhood, but do what feels best to you, no matter what other people think you should do. At the end of the day, your gut feeling matters most. It's good and fine and recommended to consider the advice of people you trust, but never ignore your instincts.

Practice the smile and nod. Again, this skill will serve you well for years to come. When someone offers you advice that goes against every fiber of the parent you want to become, just smile and nod and tell them, "Thanks. I'll consider that." It's not a lie. You just considered it, and it's the worst idea ever, so you threw it into the trash can in your brain.

Consider why the advice is coming from that person. Parenthood is so deeply personal, and it changes all parents in ways we can't begin to quantify. Each bit of advice you will get is coming at you through a lens of that person's unique experience. That's not to say it's bad or good, but consider the source. Your sister may be urging you to "just go ahead and schedule the C-section" because she wound up having an emergency C-section, but your experience isn't going to be the same as hers. Certainly consider her advice, but also consider what she has experienced that has shaped that advice.

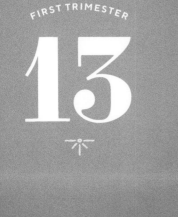

13

EAT WHAT YOU CRAVE, EXCEPT DIRT

*T*his may sound like I'm advising you to pig out and pack on the pounds. That's not what I'm getting at! However, for many of us, it's hard to eat during the first trimester, which brings me to my philosophy of eat what you crave *and* what will stay down.

Although I was grateful I didn't have to deal with vomiting, I did experience extreme food aversions and bizarre cravings (see page 60) during the first trimester of my pregnancies. Some days, it was all I could do to get a few crackers into my stomach. Don't freak out if your diet in the first trimester looks less like a healthy food pyramid and more like a bowl of noodles and cheese with a side of salty tears.

Try graham crackers, saltine crackers, dry unsweetened cereal (like Cheerios), plain bagel chips, lightly salted potato chips, or, of course, whatever you are craving.

If you are one of the lucky ones who doesn't have a volatile relationship with food in the first trimester, enjoy! Treat yourself to nutrient-rich salads, smoothies, and that pregnancy favorite, ice cream. Go to your favorite restaurant. Bonus points if it's really fancy and there's no way you're going to take a baby there.

Generally, try to be smart and mindful about what you eat. As always, listen to your doctor or midwife's advice about what to include and not include in your diet. But, most importantly, try not to let food stress you out.

JUST EAT IT

Kim Borchet, doula

Don't worry too much about what you're eating if you're sick. If you have pregnancy sickness, the most important thing is to eat whatever will stay down AND follow your cravings. If you are craving something specific, it is likely your body's way of telling you that you are lacking a certain mineral. You can focus more on healthy eating in the second and third trimesters.

COPING WITH UNUSUAL CRAVINGS

Okay, here's something that's totally bizarre, and it happened to me three out of four pregnancies: I craved rocks, sand, gravel, and cement! It's called "pica," and it's not super common, but I know enough women who have experienced this that I lobbied my editors to include this note.

According to my medical providers, the suspected culprit was my low iron levels. I had to take additional iron supplements while pregnant. I also ate real food that gave me the same texture or flavor that I was craving. For example, when I was craving grout—yes, that is a thing I just admitted—Home Depot was as tempting as any buffet. At that point, I learned to mix crushed graham crackers with frosting and ate it from a spoon. When I was craving dirt, I found that the texture and earthy flavor of raw walnuts came close.

According to AmericanPregnancy.org, some other pica cravings include burned matches, stones, charcoal, mothballs, ice, cornstarch, toothpaste, soap, sand, plaster, coffee grounds, baking soda, and cigarette ashes. This is one of those instances when you should probably avoid giving in to eating the one thing you're craving, except maybe ice. I know a lot of pregnant women love a good cup of ice. But be careful. According to Benito Benitez, DDS, MSD, "Chewing on ice can lead to chipped or cracked teeth, damage to existing dental work, and sore jaw muscles."

If you're experiencing any nonfood cravings, it's important to let your medical provider know so they can determine if there is anything missing from your diet that needs to be supplemented.

14

START FILLING YOUR PIGGY BANK

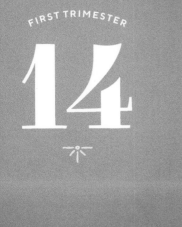

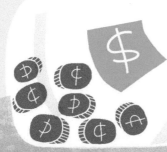

*N*ot shocking news: Babies cost money. If the thought of giving birth isn't nearly as scary to you as buying everything you need to take care of baby, take a deep breath. Time is on your side. However, it's definitely smart to start planning and saving what you can today, so you don't have to stress as much about money when you can no longer see your toes.

List it out. Make a list of the most expensive and essential items you'll need by the time baby gets here, like a crib, car seat, and stroller. Determine how much money you'll need to save to purchase those items, taking into account any offers from family and friends to gift them to you. Then schedule when you'll buy them. It's good to have the car seat and a safe space for baby to sleep at least a month before your due date.

Buy diapers in advance. Grab a box (in varying sizes) each time you grocery shop. This will help you create a diaper stash while you get used to budgeting for a larger grocery bill. Keep the boxes sealed and the receipts taped to them. There's a small chance your baby could have a reaction to the brand of diapers you purchased, or they may grow out of some sizes faster than others. Purchase from stores that will allow you to return unopened boxes.

Throw your beer and wine money onto a gift card. Take whatever money you used to spend on happy hour or stocking your wine cabinet at home, and put it on a gift card each time you shop. Save these cards to purchase baby essentials toward the end of your pregnancy.

Sign up for cash-back programs. Some websites (like ebates.com) reward you when you shop. You're bound to make more purchases now that you're expecting another person to join your family, so you may as well take advantage of these programs. Or, if you're disciplined with money, use credit cards that offer cash-back incentives to purchase baby items.

Shop secondhand. Remember that even though babies cost money, they don't have to break the bank. Consignment shops and online and offline garage sales are your friends. Recycling baby gear and baby clothes is better for your wallet and better for the world. This is the time to hit up all those well-meaning friends and relatives who have had kids recently and might have good-condition gear to give or loan.

All babies really *need* is a safe place to sleep, a safe car seat, food, diapers, clothes, and a way to be carried—either a stroller or a baby carrier.

YOUR EMERGENCY FUND

Molly Stillman, mom of two and blogger at Still Being Molly

The biggest thing we've learned as parents is that having kids means there will be unexpected expenses, and being prepared and equipped to handle it with an emergency fund when those expenses arise is so important. An emergency fund should be able to cover about three to six months of expenses. Don't let the weight of that number overwhelm you. . . . Just start somewhere and focus on saving little by little. Look at your monthly budget, allocate 5 to 10 percent for savings, and build from there.

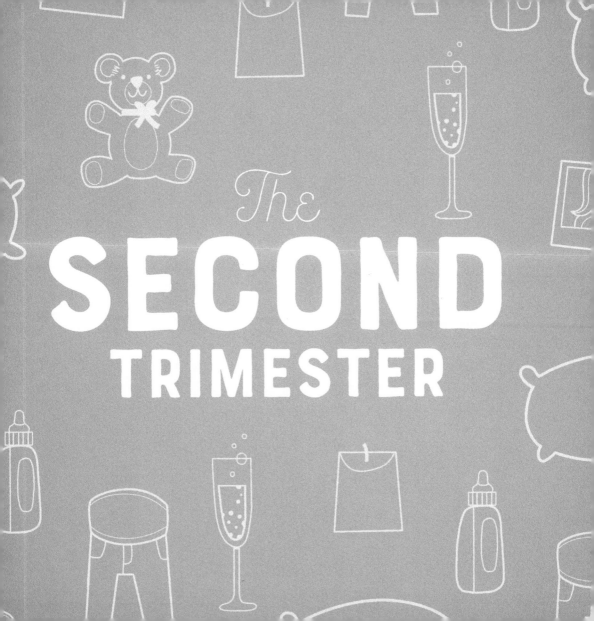

The
SECOND
TRIMESTER

They're amazing.
They've tripled in size.
I was a 34A. Now I'm a 36C.
I'm so excited! Without
being an a-hole, I have to
say, I love being pregnant.

Mila Kunis

*L*et's hear it for the girls! And by girls, of course, I mean your ample breasts. While we're at it, let's also do a happy dance for your belly that's on the verge of popping right out there and looking super adorable. The second trimester is here, and it is good, or it should be shortly. Sometimes it takes an extra week or two for any first-trimester feelings of frump and morning sickness to go away, but hope and a better relationship with food are on the horizon!

By now, you've made it through a few prenatal appointments and an ultrasound or two. It's possible you became a pro at adeptly throwing up in traffic. I'm happy to tell you that this trimester's to-dos are more about fun and less about how to survive on mashed potatoes and Sour Patch Kids.

The second trimester brings with it a resurgence of energy, and you can actually put some of that energy to use before you get super big in the third trimester. So we're going to balance doing the fun stuff with doing some important (but still mostly fun) stuff.

If you're doing a baby registry, you should create it this trimester, and whatever research you managed to do during the first trimester should help make it an easy process. And then you can relax with a mocktail and start a memory box for your baby. This is also the time to begin researching pediatricians and birthing classes.

You can also take a break and take your mind off all things baby and pregnancy—go enjoy a pre-baby vacation (babymoon), a fancy dinner, or a night out on the town. It still counts, even if you fall asleep at 8:30.

These weeks are often when most moms feel their best and feel that they look their best. You'll finally fill out some actual maternity clothes and still be able to do a workout routine. If your skin broke out in the first trimester, there's a good chance it will start to clear up now. Your nails and hair will be fierce soon if they aren't already, thanks to the hormones and prenatal vitamins.

You may really start to feel a connection with your baby this trimester. If you opt to find out the sex, that typically happens around the 18- to 20-week mark, though some of you may find out earlier. Baby really starts to move and kick around the same time. It's so extraordinary to finally feel proof of life in there!

You may find that your sex drive is off the charts. In fact, you might not be able to fit in all of these second-trimester to-dos because you'll be busy to-doing some other things in the bedroom.

When many people envision a gorgeous, happy, pregnant woman, they are thinking of one in her second trimester. So, welcome to what may be the best days of your pregnancy—you glow, girl!

15

RESEARCH AND ENROLL IN A

BIRTHING CLASS

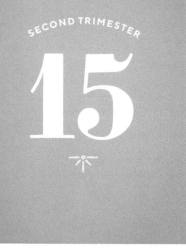

*A*t the beginning of the first trimester, you may have had to think a bit about what kind of birth you thought you wanted in order to find the right medical provider. I hope you've found a practice that is a great fit for you, whether it's an OB-GYN practice, a midwife, or a midwife who works alongside an OB-GYN.

Now, for the next "This is is getting real" task—find a birthing class. These can take as long as 6 to 12 weeks to complete, and you'll want to be sure you finish the class before you go into labor, so even though it may seem a bit early, now is actually a great time to get moving on this.

The best way to narrow down which birthing class is right for you? Start where you did when you found the best medical provider for you, and think about what kind of birth you hope to have. Do you dream of having a med-free birth, or a birth with few interventions? Then I recommend taking a birthing class that will educate you and your partner on the stages of labor and how to work your way through each one.

The Bradley Method, Hypnobabies, and Birthing From Within are all popular courses that coach parents with the goal of a med-free or low-intervention labor and delivery. These courses can mean a big time commitment, so it's important to find one that's accessible and works with your schedule. These classes range from 6 weeks to 12 weeks long, and each class can take up to three hours. For that investment of time, however, you will learn a lot about your body, your baby's development, the stages of labor, how to naturally ease labor pain, and how to prepare physically and mentally before you go into labor. You may be assigned books to read and homework between classes, like practicing relaxation techniques. Such classes will equip you with priceless tools for feeling in control and knowledgeable about childbirth—and give you a much higher chance for a med-free birth than those who don't attend such courses.

Lamaze is probably what most people think of when they imagine a birthing class. Lamaze does teach that signature breathing that we've seen portrayed in movies, but it's not just about that. Similar to the classes we just discussed, Lamaze also teaches moms how to move, use relaxation and massage, and even incorporate water to work through labor pains. This method focuses on empowering mothers to make informed choices, and is neutral about the use of pain medications such as an epidural.

If you want to give birth in a hospital and you plan to ask for an epidural as soon as possible, or if you're scheduled to have a C-section, you will likely be fine taking the birthing class offered by your hospital. That said, it doesn't hurt to take a class that offers more than you think you'll need, because, well, it's hard to know what you'll need. Some moms who planned to get an epidural ASAP never got one because their labor progressed faster than they expected!

YOU CAN FIRE
YOUR MEDICAL PROVIDER

I truly hope you are settled in with a medical provider you like and trust by now. But if you aren't and if you don't feel like your medical provider is a good fit for you, I encourage you to look into other options. You have the right to fire them!

I left my first OB at 20 weeks pregnant with my first baby and went on to have a positive pregnancy and birth experience with a group of midwives. I'm so glad I recognized when I did that the provider was not the person I wanted to help me deliver my baby.

I'm not saying that you should take this decision lightly, but trust your gut if you don't feel supported. If leaving the medical provider is not an option, look into hiring a doula. You don't have to have a med-free birth for a doula to help you. A doula is trained to provide any kind of support you need, from the physical aspect to the educational and emotional aspects. She can advocate on your behalf while you labor, and keep your specific needs in mind.

I encourage you to remain flexible, listen to your heart, and don't be afraid to advocate for yourself.

16

UP YOUR MAMARAZZI GAME

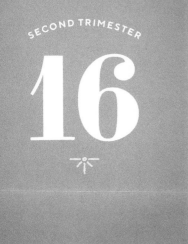

I've never met a parent who didn't cherish beautiful photos of their baby. In the olden days, like when I had my first baby in 2008, you couldn't get beautiful photos with something as simple as a phone. You had to have what I call a "fancy camera" back then, or know or pay someone who did.

From the time my first baby was born to the time my fourth was born, technology advanced. Even though I have that fancy camera now and know how to use it, it's not necessary in order to get beautiful photos of my kids. I think our generation of parents will be the first to have *more* photos and videos of each subsequent child, not fewer, because technology is continually making photography more accessible.

I love teaching parents how to get great pictures of their babies with just their phones and a couple of cheap or free apps. Here are my favorite tips:

Stock up on white bedsheets and plenty of beautiful baby blankets. White is always a lovely, neutral backdrop, and it's especially on trend right now. We spend so much time in bed with newborn babies that it's an easy spot to snap a lot of pictures in those early days. When you want to get away from white (or if you need to cover up the scene of a recent diaper blowout because you're too exhausted to change your sheets—ha, don't judge, it happens) you can layer on a colorful muslin blanket or a stretchy printed swaddle. These also make better backdrops than carpet when you take pictures on the floor.

Learn where the light is in the rooms you'll spend the most time in. The key to beautiful, crisp photos is loads of natural light (avoid using a flash). Although lighting will change with the seasons and the position of the sun, look at how the light comes into your bedroom, the baby's room, or any room you'll spend a lot of time in. Notice the shadows when you open the blinds. For the best lighting, you'll want indirect light and no harsh shadows. If the sun is shining directly into your windows at a certain time of day, look for a pocket of the room that is not in the path of the sun's rays as they come through your windows. If you don't get much light in that space, your white sheets will help. White reflects the most light, brightening up your space.

Begin playing with photo editing apps. Look for apps that let you edit the photo before you apply a filter to it. I love a good filter as much as any millennial, but remember that they may make your photos look dated in the future. And, if you're not careful, a filter can do funny things to the color of your baby's skin and hair. Instead, start by adjusting the brightness, exposure, and contrast. Then play with filters, but remember that you don't have to use them at full strength. Always keep an eye on the color of your subject's skin so it remains as natural as possible.

Look into digital photo and video storage options. Now is a great time to figure out how and where you're going to store and back up all the photos of the World's Cutest Baby. Set up a system to remove photos and videos from your phone or other cameras as your storage fills up, without having to worry about losing them forever, such as downloading them in batches to your computer each month and uploading them to an online cloud backup. Services that auto-tag faces, locations, and backgrounds will make it easier to find specific pictures in the future instead of having to scroll through thousands to find that one picture of your baby's first taste of peas.

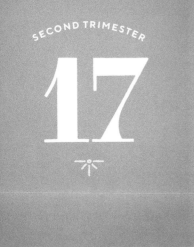

17

BEGIN A MEMORY BOX

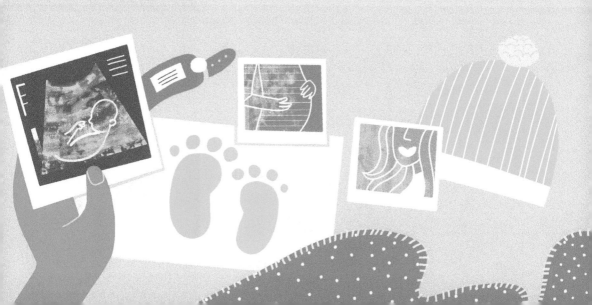

*D*on't overthink this one. I'm not asking you to decoupage or paint anything. Simply find a sturdy box with a tight-fitting lid. I recommend one that's clear plastic so it's easy to see what's in it, and not so big that it will be cumbersome once full. This will be hub central for stuff you want to save for your baby, and I encourage you to start now.

Some things you may want to put in it while you're pregnant:

— Baby shower and congratulations cards
— Ultrasound photos and video on disc or USB
— Copies of any maternity photos or belly photos
— Letters to baby
— Takeout menus with your cravings and favorite meals circled

This box will really come in handy after the baby is born. You'll have a designated space to store stuff all ready to go, meaning you won't have a pile of sentimental things to sift through by baby's first birthday.

Don't be tempted to fill the box right away. Give yourself a limit and determine how long this box should last. For me, I get a new not-so-big plastic box for each kid every three to four years. These boxes start out housing tiny baby mementos and graduate to storing pre-school artwork and elementary school report cards and homework.

I like to keep one box in baby's closet, easily accessible. I just toss things in there when I'm in a rush. As it fills up, I go through it, giving myself permission to throw out anything that doesn't seem as special anymore. I store clothes in large zip-top storage bags, and place photos, footprints, ultrasound pictures, and newspaper clippings in acid-free photo boxes to prevent fading and yellowing. I label the box with the child's name and the years the contents span. Then I put that box into a dry, dark place, like an attic or under a bed, and get a new box ready to go.

In a perfect world, you have time to meticulously put together a baby book. I wish you better luck than I had with this! But, if the baby book thing falls apart, at least you already have this system going for you. The key is to use it early and often. Don't put off going through cards that come in and clothes they outgrow. Decide right then what to save, and let go of any guilt over giving away or recycling the rest.

When you are thinking of what to save, consider this: This collection is ultimately going to be passed on to your child when they are an adult. Will what you give them be a burden or a joy? Are they going to need a U-Haul to haul away all the plastic boxes you've filled? You will find a balance between sentimentality and good sense.

Treasures that you may want to store after baby is born:

- Hospital footprints
- Hospital bracelets
- Umbilical cord remnant
- Baby's first hat and blanket
- A couple of tiny outfits they quickly outgrew
- A list of gifts people have given
- A copy of baby's birth announcement
- A newspaper from the day baby is born

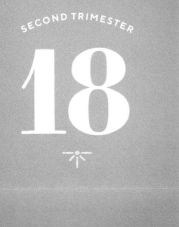

18

GET A LITTLE SWEATY

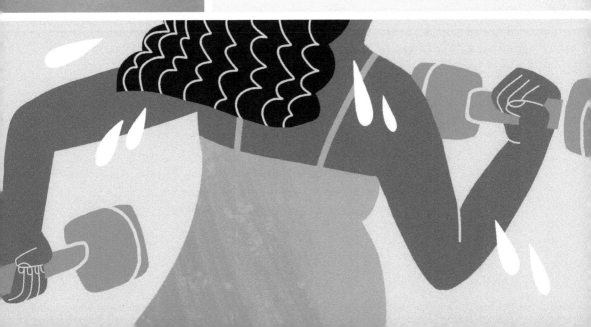

You're probably starting to feel more human, and perhaps also starting to look like you're growing a human. Take advantage of your second-trimester energy by getting into (or back into) an exercise routine—just be sure it takes into account your growing belly and loosening joints.

There are countless benefits to staying physically active while pregnant. Yes, it will likely help you keep your weight gain under control, but it can also help prevent or relieve back pain, prevent constipation, lower your blood pressure, improve your mood, and help prepare you for an easier labor.

Remember that labor is, well, LABOR. It's hard work. Personally, I always feel like I ran a marathon the day after I have a baby—and I've run two marathons, so that's not just a figure of speech. I'd never want to show up to the start of a marathon after nine months of no physical activity. Conversely, you don't have to jump into anything super intense to reap the benefits of exercise while pregnant. These are some popular pregnancy workouts that you can ease into:

Swimming or water aerobics. Being in water is especially blissful when you feel eight years pregnant and the water helps keep you upright and feeling light. The only caveats: Breathe consistently and don't hold your breath for extended periods of time.

Yoga or barre. Both of these low-impact activities can help keep you flexible and minimize back pain. You can find prenatal classes for these (a great way to meet other mamas if you haven't done that yet), but most yoga and barre class instructors will also be able to teach you pregnancy modifications during regular classes.

Light weight training. You don't have to forgo weights while pregnant, but consult your medical provider about how much you're lifting, and always keep your posture in mind to protect your back.

Walking or jogging. This may be the simplest way to ease into a pregnancy workout routine. Simply walk for 10 to 30 minutes a few times a week, and then build up from there if you'd like.

Avoid anything that involves the full use of your abs, like sit-ups or double-leg raises, and don't do any exercises that require you to lie flat on your back. Also stay away from activity that is high impact or poses a high risk of falling. Stop if you feel dizzy, or if you experience any vaginal bleeding. According to certified nurse midwife Jeanean Carter, "In the case of bleeding, stop exercise whether bleeding is painful or not. All bleeding should be reported to your health care provider. Not all bleeding means there is a problem, but it still may require treatment." As always, chat with your medical provider about your exercise plan.

KEEP IT COMFORTABLE

Jenny Bradford, yoga instructor and mom of three

I like the guideline that whatever level of activity you are accustomed to you are welcome to maintain, but you wouldn't use pregnancy as a time to start new or more aggressive activities. Walking is accessible to everyone! And most women have sciatica pain or some kind of low-back issues, so Cat Cow can feel great for spinal flexibility.

HOW TO DO A CAT COW: Find a padded and stable surface on the floor, like a yoga mat or a carpet. Get on all fours with your hands placed below your shoulders, and your knees below your hips. Your arms should be straight but relaxed. Take a deep breath, then as you exhale, push your back up to the ceiling, bring your chin to your chest, and look at your belly. Your back should be nice and round. This is Cat. When you inhale, gently drop your pelvis and belly and lift your head up. This is Cow.

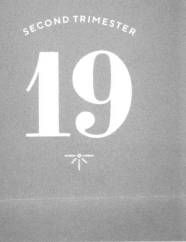

19

ENJOY A MOCKTAIL

A lot of moms completely lose the desire to have an adult beverage when morning sickness sets in. But when those clouds part in the second trimester, some of us really start to miss our happy hour faves. Whether you enjoyed cocktails prior to pregnancy or not, mocktails are a fun way to treat yourself while pregnant and after—no special occasion required. Here are a few of my favorite recipes.

Apple Cinnamon Mockscow Mule

Even if you don't have a copper mug lying around, you can still make this in a simple cocktail glass. The apple cider and cinnamon give it a nontraditional twist and make this a festive drink for holiday parties.

Ice

¼ to ½ lime

8 ounces ginger beer

4 ounces apple cider

Pinch ground cinnamon, for garnish

1 thin slice apple, for garnish

1. Fill a mug halfway with ice, then squeeze the lime over the ice.
2. Pour in the ginger beer, followed by the apple cider.
3. Sprinkle cinnamon on top, and garnish with the apple slice.

Faux Rosé All Day

This one is great to remember when you're out at brunch with your girlfriends. Any bartender should be able to throw this together for you.

3 ounces grapefruit juice

6 ounces club soda

1 to 2 tablespoons grenadine syrup

1. In a champagne flute, add the grapefruit juice, followed by the club soda.
2. Add the grenadine syrup and gently stir with a cocktail straw.

Beer Belly Rita

I don't know about you, but when I'm pregnant in the summer, I want a beer and I want a margarita—bad. This is my go-to hot-weather mocktail. Note that nonalcoholic beer still has a very small amount of alcohol in it—less than 0.5 percent. You can substitute lime-flavored sparkling water if you want to steer clear of alcohol altogether.

1 wedge lime, plus ½ lime

Kosher salt, for the glass

Ice

6 ounces nonalcoholic beer

6 ounces limeade

1. Rub a lime wedge around the rim of a glass.
2. Pour kosher salt on a plate in a thin layer. Flip the glass over and press the rim into the layer of salt.
3. Fill the glass halfway with ice. Pour in the nonalcoholic beer, followed by the limeade.
4. Squeeze the ½ lime on top, and gently stir.

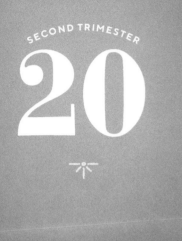

SECOND TRIMESTER

20

BEGIN TO
RESEARCH
& INTERVIEW
PEDIATRICIANS

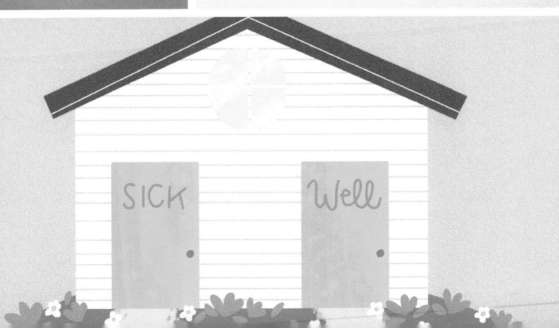

*Y*our baby's pediatrician is going to be a big part of your life, especially for baby's first years. To start your search, find someone who is easy to get to and covered by your insurance. Once you've established that, the doctor should also be easy to make appointments with and someone you personally get along with and feel at ease with, and someone who aligns with your principles and parenting style.

Begin by gathering a list of pediatricians within a reasonable drive of your home who are covered by your insurance company. Websites like Healthgrades.com can be helpful, as they provide user ratings of doctors, wait times, and office staff. Better yet, if you are friends with any local parents, or in parenting groups with any of them, ask if they have any insight or experience with any of the pediatricians on your list. Based on their feedback, you may eliminate some pediatricians and move others to the top of your list.

Next, look at the practices' websites. There, you should be able to get answers to the following questions (a quick call to speak with a receptionist should fill in any remaining gaps):

- What are their hours of operation?
- Are they open on weekends, and if so, do they see only sick patients?
- What is their cancellation policy?
- How do they handle emergencies?
- Will you see the same doctor each time, or is there a team that works to see all patients?
- Do they offer a free consultation?

Finally, narrow the list down to your top two or three offices, and call to schedule appointments. Some offices may charge for this, and your insurance is probably not going to cover it, so ask about and plan for that ahead of time.

By the time you get to the interview process, what you're really looking for is a connection with that doctor and practice. If you're up to it, ask other patients what their experience has been like while you're in the waiting room. And while you're there, look to see (or ask) if there is a separate waiting area for sick patients.

Once you're face-to-face with the doctor, ask the questions that are important to you. You may want to know how they feel about extended breastfeeding or formula feeding. You may want to know their policy on vaccinations. You may want to know their philosophy on infant sleep. Their answers will be important, but the way the doctor engages with you could be the most important.

Don't be afraid to ask the doctor if they are parents, but also don't count them out if they aren't. Two of our favorite pediatricians didn't have kids. What mattered most was the way they engaged with us. They were always attentive and never dismissed our concerns.

If your chosen pediatrician doesn't have rights at your delivering hospital, the hospital will assign you a pediatrician who will perform a checkup within 24 hours. You can have that information sent to your pediatrician, who will typically see your baby about three to five days after birth.

THE DOUBLE DOWN LOW

Beki Baker, mom of twins

Parents of multiples should consider the following factors when selecting their pediatrician: location, convenience, separated sick and well areas, working elevators, halls and waiting areas wide enough for large strollers, and friendly staff who return calls in a timely manner. Why? Multiples are often preemies, which means they have underdeveloped immune systems. Also, they share each other's illnesses pretty much every time.

Parents of multiples will be headed to the pediatrician more than average parents. Find a pediatrician close to home you love and trust because you're likely going to be seeing a lot of each other.

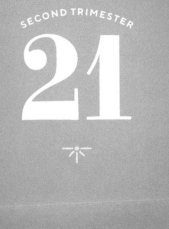

SECOND TRIMESTER

21

SHOP FOR ACTUAL MATERNITY CLOTHES

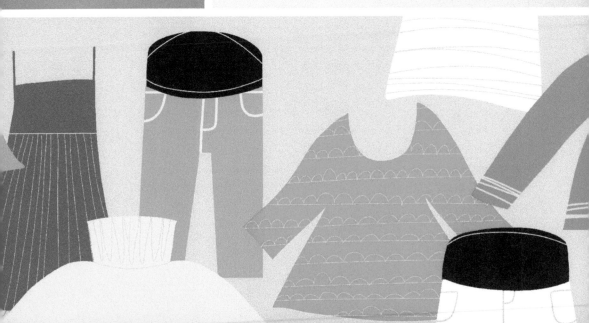

*N*ow for what I consider the fun phase, when it finally looks like there's a baby in your belly and not an overstuffed burrito. Those transition clothes you stocked up on in the first trimester are probably starting to stretch to their limit. It's time to get you some real maternity clothes!

In theory, this should be super fun, right? What woman wouldn't want an excuse to buy an all-new wardrobe? But it can be pricey as well as overwhelming, especially if you're not comfortable with your changing shape. Here are some pointers to guide you in buying or borrowing.

Everyday Basics. Start by looking through your closet to see what you have that still fits and may fit for a while longer. Items like cardigans, kimonos, oversized shirts, stretchy T-shirt dresses, and even some low-rise yoga pants could see you through most of your pregnancy. Pull those to the front of your closet, then look at where you might need to fill in some gaps.

If you are a jeans and T-shirts kind of gal, you will not regret invest-ing in at least one pair of great maternity jeans. If leggings are more your jam, there are a ton of maternity legging options. These are also great for extending the life of dresses you may already have, helping them work as tunics. Any jeans or leggings with a high waist will also work well as a fourth-trimester transition piece, so keep that in mind when you consider your investment.

Extra-long tank tops can help stretch the life of those pieces you already have, like cardigans and kimonos. Bonus points for tanks that are made specifically to support your growing belly or are nursing friendly (anything you can pull your boob out of comfortably).

Wear to Work. If you're dressing for the office, stick with a few neu-tral pieces, like a maternity pencil skirt, maternity slacks (remember, you'll get extra wear out of these post-pregnancy if they have a high waist) and a couple of blazers in a bigger size than you wore pre-pregnancy. Then switch up a few inexpensive maternity T-shirts and blouses to keep the ensemble looking fresh. Accessorize with neck-laces and scarfs you already own.

Dress Up. You'll probably have at least one dressy event between now and baby's arrival. If the thought of buying a dress just for a one-time wear annoys you, check with friends to see if they have a dress you can borrow, or check out online rental options. Dresses that can be dressed up or down are great wardrobe staples to have. I find that jersey material dresses are more comfortable than anything else, especially toward the end of a pregnancy. Pair them with flip-flops in the summer, or layer with leggings and cardigans when it's cooler outside.

You may very well have friends and family who are looking to give away (or cut you a great deal on) their maternity clothes. My sister's friends have a trunk of traveling maternity clothes that bounce from one pregnant mom to the next. A lot of moms are so done with their maternity clothes after baby comes that they'll beg you to take them before they light them on fire. If you can't find any for free, you can definitely find bags and boxes of them for cheap on eBay, Craigslist, or the Facebook Marketplace.

MATERNITY STAPLES

Valeria Rowekamp, mom of three and fashion blogger at Charmed Valerie

Don't go crazy buying tons of maternity clothes. Just focus on the staples you'd normally wear, and find maternity versions of those in colors and styles that play well together. Check out Pinterest for maternity capsule wardrobe ideas. I found my favorite pieces at baby and kid consignment stores, the clearance sections of big maternity retailers, and Target. Also, you can use bra-back extenders, belly bands, hair ties through your pants buttons, and other hacks to extend the life of your regular clothing through pregnancy and postpartum.

BUYING UNDIES
THAT FIT

While we are on the subject of buying clothes, let's not neglect how important it is to get bras and underwear that fit and feel good. No pregnant woman deserves to walk around with underwires digging into her sideboobs and a constant wedgie!

You can buy maternity underwear, or you can just get some in a bigger size than you usually wear. Look for full-coverage cheeks (or if you're into thongs, then just get those), and make sure they're low-cut to accommodate your growing belly. Also, there's a lot of moisture hanging out down there now, so it's super important they are breathable. Cotton is a safe bet. You'll want the crotch to be wide enough to stick a panty liner to because of all that moisture I just mentioned, and because sneezing and peeing yourself is about to become a thing.

As for bras, you might be tempted to jump into buying nursing bras if you plan to breastfeed, but I actually think you should wait until after your baby is born to buy any structured nursing bras (though you could get sports-bra-style nursing bras now that have more give). Your breasts are going to change in size and shape—a lot—between now and the time your milk comes in. Instead, simply get fitted for a regular bra in your current size. Then get some stretchy, low-front, V-neck, or cross-front sports or yoga bras. These work okay for breastfeeding since you can pop a boob out the top.

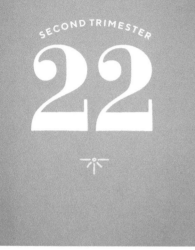

22

SAVOR
YOUR CHILD-
FREE DAYS

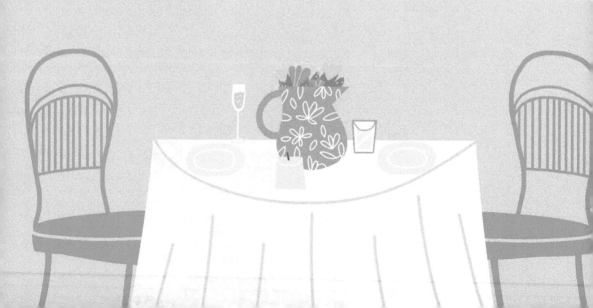

*L*et me begin with this: **I am not saying that** after you have a baby you'll never be able to do fun things again. I'm also not saying you can't do the things I'm about to tell you to do when you have a baby in tow. I'm just saying . . . you're going to have a baby. And once you have a baby, everything gets a bit more complicated. That is just a fact.

So enjoy this little pocket of time in your pregnancy before you get super big and perhaps uncomfortable. Do any or all of this stuff, and anything else you truly enjoy that may become more complicated once your baby arrives.

Go see movies and plays. Indulge in popcorn and enjoy not having to worry if your baby is going to start crying and cause you to miss the ending.

Go to music festivals and concerts. Take it all in with no distractions, from great seats or lawn seats, while you don't have to stress about a toddler running into the crowd. You can certainly bring your baby to these at some point, but you'll probably want to wait until they are old enough to wear protective headphones if it's loud.

Go out to eat! Goodness, eat at all the fancy restaurants you can, and think of me and my four children . . . I miss fancy restaurants that don't serve chicken nuggets.

Window-shop. Take a leisurely walk through stores that have expensive and breakable things at kneecap level.

Start a project and then actually finish it. Maybe make something for the baby's room, bake and decorate an elaborate cake, or cook a dinner that takes hours and leaves you feeling like a Top Chef.

Go dancing. Get dressed in your cutest maternity dress or jeans and heels and head to a bar or a club. Dance, laugh, stay up as late as you can (which probably isn't that late these days, and that's okay).

Go on a babymoon. That's like a honeymoon before you have a baby. This doesn't have to be to an exotic island. You could book a hotel for one night in your city. Heck, it doesn't even have to be with your partner. Whether you go with someone or by yourself, enjoy an escape and soak up the silence. Read a book and relax. That's the whole point.

Be intentional about relaxing and taking a break from all the stuff there is to do before you have a baby. If you want to take full advantage of a final escape before baby arrives, WEAR WHITE.

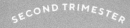

SECOND TRIMESTER

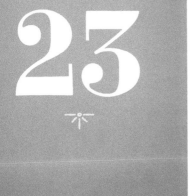

23

REGISTER

EVEN IF YOU DON'T WANT TO

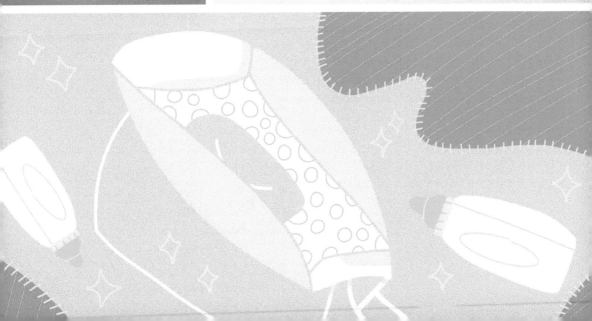

I **find that new parents either love or hate** registering for baby stuff. And if they hate it, it's often because they feel they're in over their heads. After all, how are you supposed to know what you need if you've never done this before? Registries are important, though, and it's worth your time putting something together, even if you don't feel 100 percent confident in your choices.

If you don't register, brace yourself for way too many baby blankets, infant bath towels, and other stuff that is not the car seat you really need to bring your baby home from the hospital in.

Begin with the essentials. You know you'll need a car seat, a place for baby to sleep, and a stroller and/or something to wear your baby in. All that geeking out over baby stuff you did in the first trimester should make these decisions easier.

Even as a newborn, your baby will have opinions and preferences. When it comes to bottles, I highly recommend registering for one bottle each in a few different brands, then stashing away a gift card to buy more of whatever brand your baby decides they like after they arrive. The same goes for pacifiers if you decide to use those.

People love buying baby clothes and blankets, so you may as well put some you like on your registry. Add blankets in patterns and colors that will photograph well so you can lay baby on them for Instagram-worthy pictures. Include outfits in sizes bigger than new-born and 0 to 3 months—some babies are born already too big to fit in them. If gender-neutral clothes are important, register for those, or you are bound to be inundated with pinks and blues if the sex of your baby is public knowledge.

Add boxes of disposable diapers in various sizes, and even if you don't plan on cloth diapering full time, a small stash of cloth diapers can still be useful. Nobody likes to drive to the store in the middle of the night when they suddenly realize they've run out of diapers.

The future is now, and thanks to the Internet, there are a few online baby registry services, like BabyList.com, that will bring together your registries from different stores and allow you to incorporate nontraditional baby gifts, too.

Not all things that will make life easier with baby have to come from a baby store! Here are a few of my favorite nontraditional gifts:

— Frozen meals or gift cards to your favorite restaurant that delivers
— Gift certificate for a laundry service

- Gift certificate for a housekeeper
- Professional car seat installation
- Mommy and baby yoga classes
- Gift cards to your closest drive-through coffee shop
- Easy-to-use coffeemaker and your favorite
  coffee pods

I could fill half of this book with my full registry recommendations, so instead of taking up space here, I invite you to head to BabyRabies.com/BabyRegistry to see them all. But in the meantime, here are three of my favorites:

DockATot: This is a portable place for baby to sleep—a bed that keeps baby snug. It's not a substitute for a crib, but it's a great spot to lay baby in on your bed or on the floor while you shower. The DockATot really helped our newborn sleep for long stretches, and a lot of other parents feel the same way.

Binxy Baby: Did you know you should never, ever put your baby's infant car seat on top of a grocery cart? Not even if it seems to "click" onto it. The only safe place to put a car seat in a grocery cart is inside the basket. And this can take up nearly your whole grocery cart! Binxy Baby became available only in time for me to use it with my fourth baby, and I'm straight-up mad I didn't have it with the other three! It's a baby-sized hammock for your shopping cart. It safely clips and buckles onto the cart, and you buckle your baby inside it. Then you can still fit groceries under them in the cart.

It's perfect for shopping trips before baby is old enough to sit in the front basket.

Fisher-Price Rock 'n Play: The slightly inclined and snug seat in the Rock 'n Play is a crowd pleaser on the baby circuit. It's a fantastic place for baby to nap or hang out while you make dinner or catch up on e-mails. I recommend splurging on the model that plugs into the wall, which adds the ability to vibrate, play white noise, and rock itself.

THREE THINGS YOU DIDN'T KNOW YOU NEED

Jamie Grayson, baby gear expert from The Baby Guy NYC

1. **NOSEFRIDA.** Known as the "snot-sucker," it's much more efficient and easier to clean than the blue bulb from the hospital. Sure, it's gross, but you'll get over it, because parenting can be gross.

2. **LOVE TO DREAM SWADDLE UP.** This is about as perfect of a product as you can get. Babies look REAL cute when they look like flying squirrels—and they sleep. It's also great for diaper changes.

3. **CALENDULA-BASED NIPPLE CREAM.** Lanolin is sticky and has NO skin reparative properties at all. Calendula is a flower that heals skin. Look for products by Motherlove or Earth Mama Organics. And because nipples and lips are the same skin tissue, it makes great lip balm. (#fact)

24

NOTIFY YOUR EMPLOYER
AND BEGIN PLANNING FOR MATERNITY LEAVE

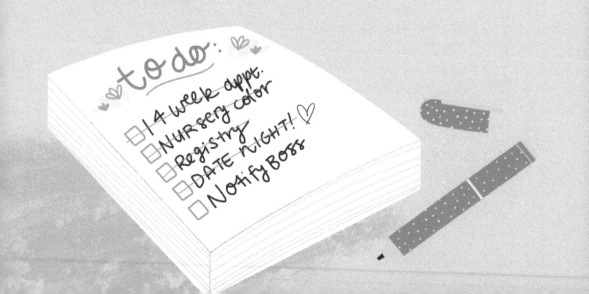

to do:
- [ ] 14 week appt.
- [ ] Nursery color
- [ ] Registry
- [ ] DATE NIGHT! ♡
- [ ] Notify Boss
- [ ]

*I*f you've been hiding your pregnancy from your employer, it's probably getting pretty difficult to camouflage your bump, so telling them could be a huge relief. But anxiety over this issue is also normal. It can be nerve-racking to give them the news with the expectation that you'll be taking time off work when your baby arrives. But there are ways to soften the blow.

Allyson Downey, founder of online platform weeSpring.com and author of *Here's the Plan: Your Practical, Tactical Guide to Advancing Your Career Through Pregnancy and Parenthood*, offers this advice:

Prepare for the discussion. Even the most effusive and supportive employer is quietly panicking inside her head, wondering, "How on earth are we going to take care of her projects while she's gone for three months?" Give her some time to react by sharing the news matter-of-factly during a regular meeting, and then say, "Over the next couple weeks, I'm going to start drafting a coverage plan, and I'd like to meet with you about it next month to talk it through and make sure nothing slips through the cracks in my absence."

Be thorough and specific in your coverage plan. Document everything on paper. One woman told me that she designed a detailed spreadsheet that included everything she was currently working on, who was running point when she was on leave, key deadlines, and what she thought the biggest risks were.

Thank your colleagues who'll be helping out. Understand that your colleagues will be carrying most of the weight while you're gone, and they may have some feelings about that. Many employers don't bother to backfill a job with a temp, and they just reallocate that job within your team. Unlike your manager, your peers haven't been taught by HR about how to react to pregnancy news, so I advise people to take the most time and care in sharing the news with their colleagues. Show your appreciation in the time leading up to your leave, make sure they feel fully prepared by the time you leave, and get as far ahead as you can in your work so the burden—and it is a burden—is lessened. When you return, share a token of gratitude (a handwritten note, pizza for the team, etc.) and go out of your way to help support *them* when they want or need to be out of the office.

Additionally, now is a good time to find out what paperwork you'll need to fill out for your maternity leave. Determine if your job offers any paid leave, if you'll be expected to use up sick days and vacation days, and if your company is legally required to offer you up to 12 weeks of unpaid leave under the Family and Medical Leave Act (FMLA). While you're at it, figure out the pumping sitch at your workplace if you plan to breastfeed and pump breastmilk when you return to work. I hope someone has gone before you and led the way to a private room (that is not a bathroom) with a table, chair, mini-fridge, and a locking door. If not, begin advocating for this.

25

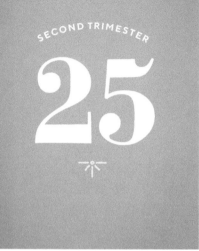

CREATE A "STORY OF US" WITH YOUR PARTNER

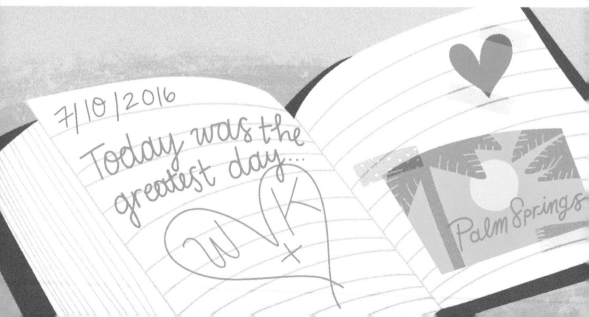

7/10/2016

Today was the greatest day...

W K x

Palm Springs

*N*aturally, so much of your focus while pregnant is on life "after baby is born." This to-do invites you to pause and celebrate life before baby comes. It also makes a great keepsake to pass on to your child when they are older—a wonderful treasure to put in their baby box.

You can be as creative and crafty with this as you'd like, but the heart of it is this: You and your partner fill a simple journal with the story of the two of you.

To start, find a journal, scrapbook, or photo album that suits your needs. Photo albums with individual 4-by-6-inch pockets are great because you can fill each pocket with either a picture or a 4-by-6-inch index card you've written on. If you choose to go the journal or scrap-book route, pick up some adhesive photo corners or photo pockets to add pictures to the pages.

Now, start at the beginning and write your story. You can either work together to tell the tale of how you met, fell in love, and had a baby, or you can each fill in a series of statements. Here are some prompts to get you going:

- We met at . . .
- Our first date was at . . . and when it was over I felt . . .
- The first time I saw your mom/dad, I felt . . .
- I knew I loved your mom/dad when . . .
- Your mom/dad's best quality is . . .
- Our favorite thing to do together is . . .
- The worst fight we ever had was about . . .
- We laughed the hardest over . . .
- We were the saddest when . . .
- The best part about loving your mom/dad is . . .
- The hardest thing we've been through is . . .
- Our favorite meal to cook or eat together is . . .
- Our best friends are . . .
- Our current hobbies include . . .
- On Friday nights we like to . . .
- We found out we were going to have a baby when . . .
- When we found out you were going to join us we felt . . .

Add pictures of you individually and as a couple. For inspiration, think of the photos you cherish of your parents, or the ones you wish you had. Reprint, or scan and print, whatever you can.

If you're going to be a single parent, tell the story of you, your strengths, your interests, and your wishes for your child and for you. No matter your story, this is a beautiful gift and a treasure for your child to enjoy and reflect on as they grow.

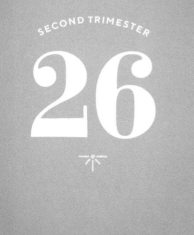

26

SOAK UP BIRTH STORIES

*F*or as long as women have been giving birth, women have been telling other women their birth stories. Each one is compelling in its own way, and no two are the same. Birth is magical like that, and I think you should absolutely soak up as many stories of that magic as you can.

Birth can also sound a little horrifying, depending on the birth stories you're hearing and reading. There's no shortage of mothers who will want to warn you or tell you about the stuff that was hard and scary from their perspective. There's space for these stories, but it's important to be intentional about the birth stories you're consuming.

Use birth stories as a tool to help you visualize and prepare for the birth you hope to have, and use them as a way to prepare for birth going differently than you have planned. Listening to or reading the birth story of a mom who had an emergency C-section doesn't mean you'll be more likely to have one, but it can help you understand what you could expect if you find yourself in that situation.

Birth stories should be positive, empowering, and moving reminders that women are powerful badasses. No matter how you plan to birth, or how you end up giving birth, YOU are going to be incredible at bringing your baby into this world. Seek out the birth stories that inform and inspire you.

You can begin by asking your friends and family who've been there to tell you their stories. If there's any part of labor and delivery that has you particularly nervous, ask them specifically about their experiences. Maybe you're afraid you won't know what a contraction feels like, or you're terrified of what will happen if you poop while pushing.

It can feel too personal asking people you actually know some of these things, though, or maybe you don't have many friends in your life who've done this before. No worries! There are plenty of other places where you can read and hear any and all types of birth stories, including blogs specifically dedicated to curating and sharing them; a basic Google search will lead you to those. Your childbirth class may even have its own online collection, or examples in the books you're reading. For an even more immersive experience, you can watch birth videos on YouTube, but I find that hearing the whole story from the mother's perspective, including her inner thoughts and feelings, gives a better, bigger picture.

My favorite way to take in birth stories is via *The Birth Hour* podcast. Podcast host Bryn Huntpalmer has recorded hundreds of mothers and fathers who tell their own unique birth stories, and these cover the entire spectrum of labor and delivery outcomes. Each episode is about an hour long, and you can listen to them for free, however you prefer to access podcasts.

SHARING BIRTH EXPERIENCES

Bryn Huntpalmer, host of The Birth Hour *podcast*

When I was pregnant with my eldest, my love of (OK, obsession with) birth stories began. I would Google "birth stories" and watch YouTube videos of births until 3:00 a.m. many nights—not exactly the healthiest practice when you are growing a human.

For other moms-to-be, I wanted it to be easier to find informative, supportive, and empowering birth stories. I spent more than a year thinking about the idea and planning for *The Birth Hour* podcast before I launched it. The podcast is a mental preparation for birth. Hearing all of the ways that birth can happen (and has happened) is a great way to get ready. When something went differently than expected, listeners have told me that they drew strength from all of these other moms' stories, knowing they were not alone. *The Birth Hour* shares all types of birth stories and doesn't promote one way of giving birth as being better than another. It's a way to come together as a community of mothers, and support each other no matter how our births go.

SECOND TRIMESTER

27

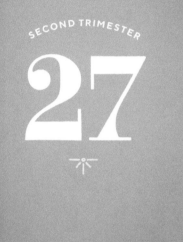

BRACE YOURSELF FOR RUDE COMMENTS

ARE YOU SURE IT'S NOT TWINS?

*A*s you near the end of your second trimester, your belly is going to begin to attract the attention of more and more people. Sometimes it's fun, or at least funny. But don't feel alone or like you're overreacting if it feels rude, awkward, or even hurtful.

A lot of people mean well when they say, "Bless your heart, you look like you're about to pop!" But hearing that when you're only 25 weeks pregnant can sting, and it doesn't matter how lovingly they meant it. Also, I'm not convinced that anyone who repeatedly asks "You sure it's not twins?" means well at all.

Sometimes the only way to get the gal in the cubicle next to you to quit asking if you're sure you got your due date right and you aren't going to have the baby tomorrow is to look her in the eye and say something snarky to her.

Keep these comebacks in mind next time someone says something that seems far from "well-meaning":

- "Twins? Oh no, I'm actually having a litter. Would you like one?"
- "Yeah, I'm reminded how huge I am every time I see myself naked in the mirror, but thanks."
- "If you think my butt has gotten big, you should see my nipples!"
- "I guess my due date could be off by three months. Maybe my water broke today. I thought I just peed my pants."
- "My doctor confirmed that I am having a boy, but I'll be sure to tell them you think they're wrong because my hips are too big. Maybe they can hire you to replace the ultrasound machine."

My favorite is the cold, hard, long stare, followed by silence or "We're keeping that to ourselves for now." Because nobody is entitled to know your due date or if you're having more than one baby and if that baby is a boy or a girl, especially not random strangers.

Now, a few of these people are going to do more than just comment—they are going to TOUCH. Some will kindly ask first. I always appreciate that, and have been known to say yes to a kind lady wanting to rub my belly. But some just reach right out there and pat you down like the TSA, and that is so not cool. This is still YOUR body! If someone touches you and you don't want them to, tell them to stop. No snarky comeback needed. "Please don't touch me," if you're feeling generous.

28

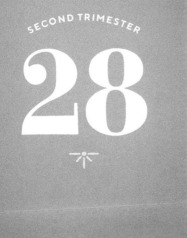

CREATE A
BIRTH PLAN

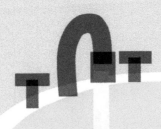

*W*HOA, whoa, no . . . what? Did I just suggest you create a birth plan? Like a plan for when this baby exits your womb, which is surely a long time from now? It may feel like you're still a long ways off from meeting your sweet peanut, but a birth plan can take a while to bring together.

What one might imagine a birth plan to be: pages of super specific requests, like what song you want playing when your baby crowns and how you'd like the room to be filled with candlelight while you push.

What a birth plan should actually be is a page where you list your most important requests, such as:

- If or when you'd like an epidural
- Whether you plan to breastfeed or bottle-feed your baby
- How you'd like to manage any pain once you have the baby

Most importantly, a birth plan should be well researched. It's important to know if your request can actually be accommodated by your medical provider, or if where you'll be giving birth has restrictions on your wishes. For example, some hospitals will allow you to labor in water, but they discourage pushing and giving birth in water. That's definitely something you'll want to know before you add "water birth" to your birth plan.

Your birth plan should also be flexible. Absolutely put safeguards in place to give you a better chance of achieving the kind of birth you'd like. It's okay to do everything you can to avoid a C-section, but it's also important to be prepared and consider how you wish to handle that situation if it does arise. It's also good to be familiar with the practices of the hospital you'd be transferred to if complications arise during a home or birth center birth.

You can arrange for a certain song to be playing, and even plan to push in a certain position, but these are small details that either won't matter or may change when you are in that moment, so don't stress over them now. Instead, begin formulating your birth plan by considering the following:

- Do you want an epidural, and if so, when?
- Do you want an IV?
- Do you want to be able to get up from your bed and change positions to work through labor pains?
- Who would you like in the room with you?
- Will you have a doula?
- Are you okay with continuous monitoring or would you prefer intermittent monitoring?

- Would you like to delay cord clamping?
- Would you like immediate skin-to-skin contact with your baby?
- Would you like to delay eye antibiotics?
- Would you like to postpone baby's first bath?
- Will you be breastfeeding?
- How would you like to be treated for pain after the baby is born?

This is not a comprehensive list, but it is a good place to start. Some medical providers will offer you a template to create a birth plan along with them. What matters most is that there's open communication beforehand.

THE TEAM PLAN

Hanan Webster, birth and postpartum doula

Creating a birth plan should be more than a Pinterest-inspired chart with your dos and don'ts for birth. It can be a great tool to have with you for your birth team and nurses at a hospital, but it's more beneficial to have continuous communication with your provider at each prenatal visit about your birth desires and preferences.

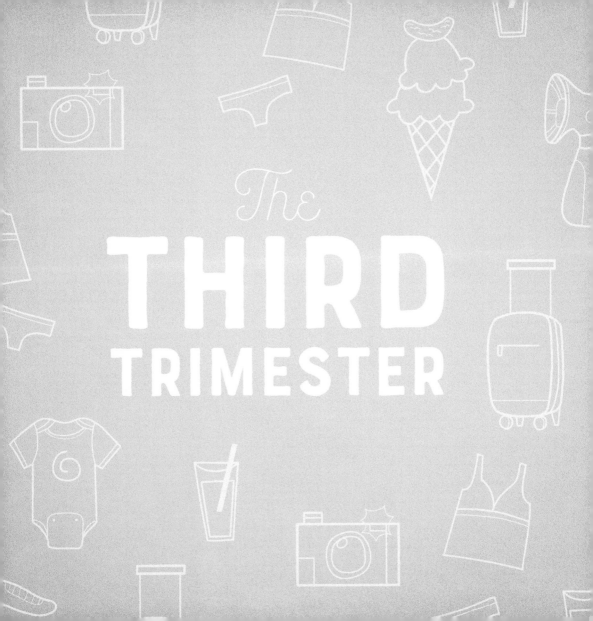

The

THIRD
TRIMESTER

When you are pregnant you can get away with a lot of sh*t. Your hormones are telling you that you are strong and sexy, everyone is scared of you, and you have a built-in sidekick who might come out at any minute.

Amy Poehler

The second trimester gave you time to get used to the idea of being pregnant, and now the third trimester is all about getting you used to the idea of becoming a mom. That little sidekick is going to be here before you know it. But also? It's going to feel like an eternity from now until the baby is born. Thanks, Parenthood Time Warp! Never change! (It never will. From now on, for the rest of your life, time will move all at once and not at all simultaneously.)

Other things happening all at once and not at all right now include everything that you feel needs to be done before you have a baby. That nesting instinct is getting really strong, but so is your urge to live in sweatpants on your couch. This is when it's key to work smarter, not harder. Prioritize what really needs to get done, and flex that self-care muscle: Ask. For. Help.

Listen, even if everything on your "This MUST get done before I have a baby" list doesn't get accomplished, it's going to be fine! What's most important is that you're listening to your medical provider and your body, and you're doing everything you can to keep yourself and your baby healthy.

This is when the focus of your pregnancy may become more about you and less about the excitement of having a baby. You're probably going to feel uncomfortable, emotional, and over-whelmed at least some of the time. It's okay to demand that your partner, your family, and your medical providers listen to you and help you find some ways to feel better and more in control.

It's common for there to be tension between pregnant moms and their partners, especially at this stage. Try to remember that while YOU are the one who's waking up every few hours to pee and enduring heartburn to end all heartburn, your partner is also trying to wrap their head around the rapidly approaching life change that awaits them. I feel confident saying that most of the fights you have now will be hilarious to you in a year. But that doesn't make them fun in the moment. I get it. It's okay to sob if your partner throws away your favorite jar of pickle juice because OF COURSE the juice is TOTALLY the best part and they're a fool for not knowing that. I'm also saying, though, that maybe you don't actually file for a divorce or move out over it.

Focus your energy this trimester on transitioning your excitement about being pregnant to making plans for becoming a parent. There are some big decisions that need to be made. Yes, nail down birth plans and baby-feeding plans, but also prepare and educate yourself in case those plans change. Basically, take control of what you can, and feel confident enough to roll with the rest.

It's not all serious these next few months, though. Even though pregnancy can start to get physically challenging now, it can also get a lot more fun if you enjoy folding tiny laundry, setting up cribs, and installing car seats. Okay, maybe "fun" isn't the word you'd use to describe all that, but it's definitely getting real and hopefully in an exciting way. Enjoy what you can. Take a lot of pictures, rock a bikini, and connect with your best friends over brunch and whine.

Feel strong, feel sexy, feel accomplished, and get ready to meet your new little sidekick!

29

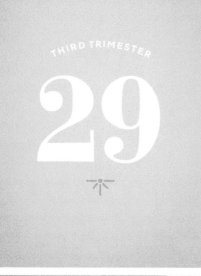

FLUFF YOUR NEST

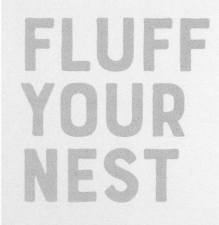

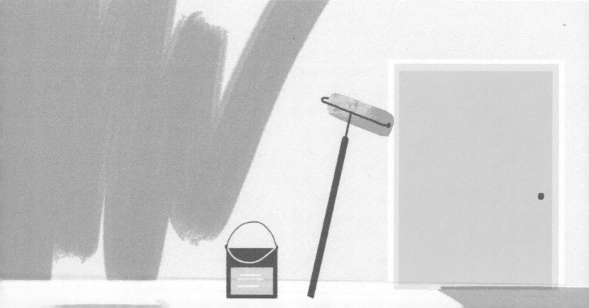

A **baby is coming! A baby is coming! This** house is not ready for a baby. These floors are not clean enough for a baby. Goodness, that closet is never going to be ready for a baby. And this Tupperware? I must find all the matching lids before I'm ever ready for a baby!

That was a not-so-dramatic reenactment of me right before having each of my four babies.

A surge of energy, coupled with increasing anticipation, can make you want to clean, organize, purge, and put in new carpet right this very minute. This is commonly referred to as "nesting." You're probably not going to have the time or money to do everything on your list. So instead of spending an entire afternoon matching your Tupperware lids and vacuuming the dust bunnies out from behind your bookshelves, here are some projects I would prioritize if the nesting urge strikes you:

Make YOUR bedroom a sanctuary. We tend to focus a lot on making baby's room beautiful and comfortable, but you will probably spend just as much time, if not much, *much* more time, in your room during the first few months. Have the carpet steam cleaned, dust the ceiling fan, maybe top the bed with a new soft blanket. Consider adding a TV if you don't have one, or a stack of new-to-you books to keep you occupied while you snuggle in with your sleeping newborn. If you have room, add a comfortable chair where you can feed and rock your baby. If you don't have them yet, be sure you get proper pillows to support your back while sitting up in bed. Make it a space you'll be happy to spend your waking hours in.

Clear visible clutter. Focus on projects that are visible to you first. Declutter counters, bookshelves, and tables. Clean and clear surfaces will help your space feel calm, because calm is a great thing to feel when you have a newborn. Don't just shove this stuff in another cabinet. Take the time to purge what you don't need anymore, and find useful and logical spots for the rest to prevent you from having to deal with the same clutter again after your baby is born.

Catch up on ALL your laundry. Baby laundry is pretty easy to get excited about, so get that out of the way, for sure. Wash, fold, hang, and put away all those ridiculously adorable baby clothes and blankets. But don't neglect your own laundry! Don't just clean (and PUT AWAY) your clothes. Clean out your drawers and closet, and organize them so you can easily find your most comfortable postpartum clothes once baby comes. If you have any pieces that need dry cleaning, do that now, too.

Finish that unfinished project. I think most of us have at least one unfinished project around the home. Perhaps there's a room you left half-painted or picture frames on the wall that don't actually have pictures in them yet. Finish that project!

The nesting instinct is strong for a lot of pregnant moms, though not all, so don't feel like you're broken if you really don't care if your newborn comes home to a house with dirty baseboards. The baby will never notice.

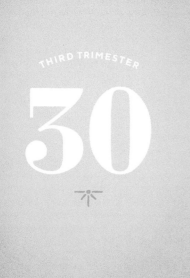

30

PREREGISTER WITH YOUR HOSPITAL OR BIRTH CENTER

LABOR and DELIVERY

*I*t's time to start thinking about the moment you'll say "it's time." If you're planning to drive to a hospital to give birth, go ahead and preregister there now while you can fill out the forms without having to stop to breathe through a contraction.

Because your medical provider has to have privileges to deliver at the hospital you go to, you've probably already chosen that hospital. Hop on over to the hospital's website and check to see if they let you preregister online. If not, call to see when you can swing by to fill out the paperwork. Be sure to bring your insurance information. This won't mean you'll pull up to the hospital in labor and be whisked into a delivery room. There will still be questions to answer when you get there, but preregistering should cut the number of questions down by quite a bit. This also gets the ball rolling with your insurance in case they require preauthorization for your stay.

While you are there, either on their website or at the hospital, find out when you can tour the labor and delivery (L&D) unit, and make a reservation for that tour if needed. If it's possible, try to do it at a time when your partner or labor support person can come with you.

It may seem pretty straightforward, but an L&D tour can help you feel more familiar and at ease with your surroundings when you're in labor, and you can use that time to ask questions, like what is their protocol for keeping babies in the L&D wing safe, and where can you find the best food at two in the morning.

If you're giving birth in a birth center that's not associated with a hospital, you're probably already seeing your midwives there and don't need to preregister or get a tour, but the next tip is for both you and hospital-bound mamas.

If you plan to get in a car to get to the place you're going to give birth, it's important to think, even if very briefly, about what you'll do if you don't make it to the hospital or birth center on time. The chance you'll give birth in your car is very small, but it does happen. Here are a couple of ways to be prepared for that tiny chance:

1. Make sure both you and your partner or labor support person have phone numbers for your provider and hospital or birth center on speed dial. Either call them to let them know you'll need immediate help upon arrival if you are in active labor, or call them AFTER you call 911 while giving birth.

2. Keep a few clean towels and baby blankets in your passenger seat, plus a couple of large trash bags. These can also be helpful if your water breaks before you get to the hospital.

STOCK UP
FOR YOUR HOME BIRTH

—⁂—

Desiree Fawn, trained doula and prenatal educator, offers the following advice for those preparing for a home birth:

Beyond the typical home birth must-haves that a care provider is going to recommend (such as awesome plastic sheets to put on your bed), here are a few other things to add to your list:

LIP BALM. Your lips will likely be super dry, no matter what season it is. Stay away from vanilla, berry, or other sweet scents—you won't want them.

STRAWS. Straws or a plastic cup with the built-in straw and lid will make it easier for you to drink no matter what position you're in (especially if you're lying down or on your hands and knees). It also makes it easy for people to help you drink.

TENNIS BALL. These are great for providing a pressure point on your back or rolling under your feet.

HOUSECOAT AND SLIPPERS WITH GRIPS. These provide a quick cover-up for warmth when you want it, and a safe way to walk around after being in the shower or birthing tub.

ICE. Fill all your ice cube trays, or buy an extra bag of ice, to keep on hand for the big day. During the last phases of labor, you'll likely want a cold cloth on your forehead or neck. Keeping a bowl with ice and facecloths close by is faster and more efficient than having someone run back and forth to hold the cloths under a cold tap.

→

FLASHLIGHT. Your caregiver will likely have one, but this is also helpful for your partner if they need to see something but you're feeling more comfortable in the dark.

RICE BAG OR ANOTHER TYPE OF HEATING BAG. This is great for your back or belly, depending on where you're feeling the contractions most. You can also squeeze the rice bag during contractions for comfort.

CRANKED-UP WATER HEATER. Whether or not you're planning a water birth, you might find it helpful to turn up the dial on your water heater. This will prevent you from running out of hot water as quickly, and it'll make sure the tank heats up faster as you use more water. Running water is a great analgesic, and if that's working for you, you'll want to stay in as long as possible. Be sure to leave a note on sinks and showers letting people know you've turned up the heat so they don't accidentally burn themselves.

31

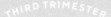

CREATE A BUMP PHOTO SHOOT

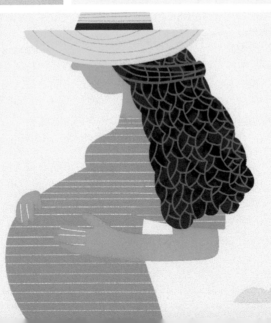

I've never met a mom who regretted taking maternity photos, but I know plenty who regret not taking them. It's time to celebrate that gorgeous bump with a photo shoot.

If you plan to hire a professional, know that most photographers recommend scheduling these photos for the beginning of your third trimester. Try to get in touch with the photographer with enough advance notice to get on their calendar in time.

Pick an outfit that makes you feel confident and beautiful. Empire-waist maxi dresses are wonderfully flattering for most body types. The fabric can hug your belly and hide your legs at the same time. Throw a flowy cardigan over it for cooler weather or if you feel self-conscious about your arms. Maternity leggings and tunics are also comfortable options that photograph beautifully.

If you feel best in your favorite maternity jeans, that works, too! Pair them with a simple, solid-color maternity T-shirt, and then jazz up the whole outfit with a statement necklace and shoes. The best part about wearing high heels for pictures is that you only have to stand in them for a few minutes at a time. Alternatively, go barefoot and show off your pedicure. Or take some boudoir shots with just your skivvies on or an artfully placed sheet or hands to cover your bits—if Demi Moore started the trend, Serena Williams made it glorious, and Beyoncé and the Kardashians broke the Internet with it, you can do it, too. You don't have to show these to anyone, but they may blow your mind in a few years. You can also take the same shot but holding your baby postpartum for a really awesome before and after.

There are so many ideas on Pinterest for cutesy or themed maternity shoots, but don't stress out or overcomplicate it. The focus should be on your belly and your face. A beautifully lit portrait in a local park can become as much a treasure to you as a staged photo of you, bare belly out, eating pickles on the floor at Target.

If you don't have the funds or the time to find a professional photographer, don't worry. Here are a few tips for getting timeless shots with a simple point-and-shoot camera or your smartphone:

Get outside about an hour before the sun sets. (You can look up exactly when the sun is going to set that day on weather.com.) Find a location with a background you like (no ugly buildings or highways in the background) that has the sun setting off to the side of you when you look at the camera.

Have your partner or whoever is taking the pictures get a lot of angles. Get some close-up shots of your hand resting on your belly and some shots of you sitting on the ground (don't forget to bring a pretty blanket!) looking up at the camera. Look away for some, look at the camera for others. Smile, don't smile. Get a lot of pictures so chances are you'll love at least a few.

Nail the silhouette shot. Stand directly between the setting sun and the photographer, and turn to the side so your full profile is showing. The sun behind you should nicely silhouette your bump.

You can then edit these photos with a photo app, such as A Color Story, Snapseed, and VSCO. Chose a filter that keeps your skin as natural looking as possible.

A SHOOT TO TREASURE

Erin Hoskins, maternity and newborn photographer at Erin Elizabeth Photography

Maternity photos are a fabulous way to remember your pregnancy. Many of my clients feel huge, uncomfortable, and not at all camera ready; however, each of them put those feelings aside and ended up absolutely treasuring those final images.

Choose timeless clothes. In 20 years, will you still love what you decided to wear? I prefer flowing dresses; movement always adds depth and beauty to images.

Pose naturally, with emphasis on the belly. I accentuate my clients' curves by having each bending her knee and keeping at least one hand on the belly for most of the session.

Above all, keep things positive. As I always say to clients, "Don't forget to look like you're happy to be having a baby!"

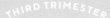

32

STOCK FOOD YOU CAN EAT WITH ONE HAND

*B*abies make you hungry, but for most new moms, it's hard to find time to sit down to three hot meals a day. Snacks are going to become life sustaining, and it's important that you're able to eat them with one hand! Why? Because you're not going to want to put your beautiful baby down, or they won't want you to put them down. Either way, lots of holding is going to happen, and you need at least one arm and hand for that.

Start stocking your pantry and refrigerator with groceries for easy one-handed snacks and meals. On the next two pages are a few of my favorite postpartum foods.

Peanut Butter Pancake Tacos

2 frozen pancakes

2 tablespoons peanut butter

1 banana, thinly sliced

¼ cup mini chocolate chips

1. Heat up the pancakes, then spread a generous layer of peanut butter on top of each.
2. Top with the sliced bananas and mini chocolate chips. Fold in half, like a taco.

Egg & Veggie Burritos

1 flour tortilla

2 eggs, scrambled

1 cup fresh spinach, sautéed
    until wilted

2 slices roasted red peppers

¼ cup crumbled goat cheese
    (see tip)

1. Put the tortilla on a plate. Top with the scrambled eggs.
2. Add the spinach and roasted red peppers, and sprinkle with the goat cheese crumbles. Fold into a burrito.

Tip: Some moms choose to limit their dairy intake while breast-feeding, especially during the first couple of months, in case their baby is lactose intolerant. Goat cheese doesn't have the same proteins as cow's milk, so it can be a good substitute when you're missing Cheddar.

Ham & Egg Cups

Baking spray

6 to 12 slices deli ham

6 eggs

1 cup fresh spinach (optional)

1 cup shredded cheese,
for topping

1. Preheat the oven to 400°F. Coat the cups of a muffin pan with baking spray. Press 1 slice of ham into each muffin cup (2 slices if very thin).
2. Crack 1 egg into each cup. Top with the fresh spinach (if using).
3. Bake for 15 to 18 minutes, or until the eggs are as done as you'd like them. Sprinkle with the shredded cheese.
4. Allow to cool for a few minutes, then use a butter knife to loosen each cup and pop the ham and egg cups out of the muffin tin.

OTHER ONE-HANDED MEAL AND SNACK IDEAS

- Smoothies
- Panini
- Grilled cheese sandwiches
- Quesadillas
- Cheese sticks
- Dried fruit
- Nuts
- Prosciutto-wrapped melon slices
- Breakfast bars
- Oatmeal cookies (oatmeal is great for your milk supply!)
- Yogurt in a tube
- Meat pies or empanadas
- Bagels and cream cheese

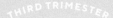

THIRD TRIMESTER

33

PREP AND STORE FREEZER MEALS

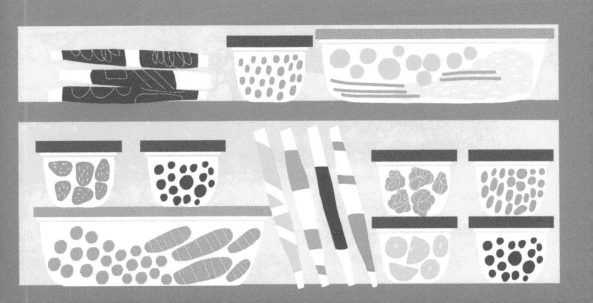

*I*t's common for people to suggest that expecting parents make freezer meals to prepare for the first few weeks after baby is born. The idea is that these are premade meals, ready to take right out of the freezer and eat. If you're on a tight budget, they can be key in keeping you well fed without spending a lot of money on delivery food or grocery store conveniences. And you can make them and freeze them ahead of time . . . like, now!

DO

- Plan to make a lot of them in one weekend instead of a few at a time. You can turn your kitchen into a meal-prep assembly line, and you'll have to clean up only once.
- Grocery shop in bulk so you can maximize money savings. Plan your meals around what's on sale and in season at the time.

- Ask friends and family to come over and help you prep the meals (or better yet ask them to make something for your freezer). This is a great way to practice asking for help!
- Look online at Pinterest or for recipes with lots of good reviews for meal inspiration, but also stick with favorites you know you'll love.

DON'T

- Don't just make a bunch of casseroles. There are many other meals you can make ahead and freeze. Try adding in some soups, wraps, burritos, pancakes, and stir-fries to keep you from feeling like you're eating various versions of lasagna for a month.
- Don't forget dessert! Make your favorite cookie dough, roll it into balls, and freeze for fast, fresh, and warm cookies on demand.
- Don't overwhelm yourself. Plan ahead, don't grocery shop and prep meals on the same day, keep it simple, and label your meals when you finish so you don't mix them up.

If prepping entire meals ahead of time doesn't work for you, you can still put a meal plan in place now by stocking your freezer with items that will help you throw together meals in less than 10 minutes. Tiffany Dahle, blogger at *Peanut Blossom*, suggests the following:

Taco feast. Season and brown batches of ground beef with your favorite taco seasoning. Freeze the batches in meal-size portions.

Keep a package of tortillas and your favorite jarred salsa in the pantry ready to go. Serve with a simple bagged salad or chips and salsa.

Bolognese sauce packets. Freeze smaller packages of meat-filled Italian Bolognese sauce and use it to top freshly prepared pasta or gnocchi. Bake a frozen garlic bread and serve with the pasta and a bag of salad.

Prepared meatballs and flavored sausages. Stock up on your favorite brands of meatballs and sausages. There are tons of delicious chicken sausage varieties available. They can quickly be browned in a skillet when you're ready to eat. Cut the sausages into slices before cooking to make it go even faster. Serve the sausages as sliders on small buns, over rice, or with pasta, along with your favorite condiments.

Veggie soup. Make a big batch of your best vegetable soup and freeze individual portions that can easily be reheated. Then stock a bag of dinner rolls in your freezer to serve with it.

DO YOUR BODY A FAVOR
THE ART OF THE PADSICLE

Okay, so you're likely to stock your freezer with food at some point during the third trimester. While you're at it, do your post-baby body a favor and make a few padsicles to have on hand.

What the heck is a padsicle? A feminine hygiene pad that you freeze, of course. If you have a vaginal birth, this is a game changer to soothe your sore lady bits and help them heal faster.

What follows here and on the next page is a padsicle DIY courtesy of Amy Morrison, founder of the blog *Pregnant Chicken.*

What You'll Need

EXTRA-HEAVY OVERNIGHT PADS. The bigger the better, because there ain't no party like thunderpad party. Try to get them without wings if you're wearing mesh underwear or boyshorts because they just get in the way.

WITCH HAZEL. Skip the alcohol. Save booze for your face bits, not your lady bits.

ALOE VERA GEL. Be sure it's unscented and free from alcohol because that would probably jack up the sting factor.

LAVENDER ESSENTIAL OIL (OPTIONAL). This helps speed healing and smells nice.

LARGE ZIP-TOP BAGS. To hold your pad stash in the freezer.

→

How To

1. Unfold your pad. If it has wings, remove the tabs, but save them because you'll need to put them back on.

2. Saturate the pad with the witch hazel (3 or 4 tablespoons) so the pad is good and soaked.

3. Pump or spoon about 2 tablespoons of aloe onto the pad.

4. Add 1 or 2 drops of lavender oil (if using).

5. Using the back of a spoon, spread the aloe and lavender evenly over the pad.

6. Gently refold your pad (reuse your wing tabs so the whole thing doesn't stick together).

7. Put your pads in the zip-top bag and pop it in the freezer.

Once you're ready to feel the "Ahhhh..." simply remove the pad from the freezer and let it thaw a bit (you want cold, not frozen, because you don't want to have to explain that kind of frostbite). Use it as you would a regular pad. These do get wet, so consider sitting on a towel or in a place where you don't mind leaving a bit of a puddle.

PREPARE FOR DOWNTIME

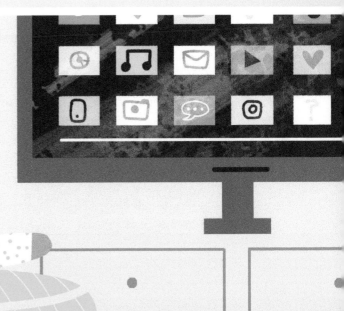

$\mathcal{H}$aving a newborn to take care of is the world's best excuse for staying in your PJs all day and accomplishing nothing other than keeping a little human alive and happy. And while that is hard work sometimes, you can do that while also binge-watching your favorite show. Life with a newborn is equal parts fun and exhausting like that.

So what are you going to do with this downtime? Let's come up with a plan!

TV Binges. To start, I suggest choosing a binge-worthy series on the streaming service of your choice. The more seasons already out, the better! You can go with a favorite, or with something that will make you feel really hip to pop culture and relevant at dinner parties that maybe you will get to attend again someday. This is one of the few times you can use parenting as a way to up your cool factor.

If you're staying home with baby while your partner works, find something you can watch all by yourself without feeling like you're cheating on them. Or watch episodes of a shared series individually with a promise that the two of you will watch the finale together.

Podcasts. You won't always be able to sit still in front of a TV. Add in some podcasts to the mix. Podcasts are great for listening to while you take long walks with baby or drive them around the block 50 times so they will nap.

Audiobooks. In theory, paper books are a great thing to plan on catching up on, but I find it hard to hold the baby and read at the same time. It's a little easier when an e-reader or tablet eliminates the pesky and surprisingly noisy task of turning a page inches away from your baby's sleeping face.

New movies. Don't count out catching movies in the theater. Once you get the hang of feeding your baby—and I don't mean that patron-izingly; there can be quite a learning curve—and once you have a good feel for when they might start to get sleepy, a dark movie theater can be a great place to take a newborn. Dress them in warm clothes and bring a blanket since it tends to get cold in those spaces, and try to sit away from other people so you won't feel self-conscious about tiny baby noises and feeding them if needed. I wouldn't recommend going to a 7:00 p.m. showing on a Friday night, or a really loud action movie, and I'd always be prepared to step out if your baby begins crying. But chances are, your baby will fall asleep and stay asleep for a good portion of the movie. They may even find the loud movie theater noises soothing. So look ahead to see what movies are coming out, and make a plan to try it out.

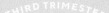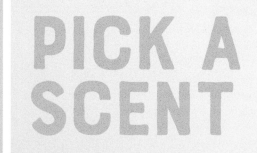

THIRD TRIMESTER

35

PICK A SCENT

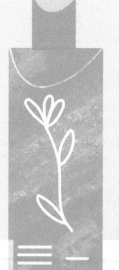

*S*mell and memory are physiologically linked. Yes, there's a perfectly good, scientific reason why the smell of freshly sharpened pencils takes you back to the fourth grade, and it's the same reason why you should pick a scent that will one day help bring you right back to the days you cradled a newborn. It has something to do with the olfactory bulb (responsible for processing smells) being close to the hippocampus (responsible for recalling memories) in your brain. Science works.

Pick a scent that you haven't already associated with anything else, and train your brain to associate it with memories of your baby.

For me, this wound up being a lightly scented baby lotion and shampoo that we used for all of our babies. Anytime I smell it, I'm immediately taken right back to those moments when I wrapped my freshly cleaned newborn up in a soft towel and covered them in lotion before I stuffed them into their PJs.

If you would rather avoid scented lotions and soaps for your baby, apply a lotion or your favorite essential oil blend to yourself. Treat yourself to an indulgent hand cream and keep it on your bedside table. Apply it each night before you put your baby to bed.

Why on earth am I telling you to do this? This is something that was suggested to me before I had my first baby, and I'm SO GLAD I did it. When you're living life with a newborn, those moments feel so raw and deep. It's hard to imagine ever forgetting them. But we do. Having a way to recall the weight of my babies' warm bodies and the softness of their skin has been such a gift. I truly hope when I'm 88 years old, I'll still recall all those moments just as easily when I smell that scent.

So spend a little time thinking about and smelling scents. Intentionally pick one you love, and one that you will be able to find years from now when you want to recall life with a newborn.

36

WEAR A BIKINI

*Y*ou are a rock star right now. Seriously. Look at you! You are growing a WHOLE OTHER PERSON. Your body is doing some incredible stuff, and you should be so very proud of it.

You're probably very visibly pregnant by now, and that's why this to-do can be so much fun. You *can* rock the heck out of a bathing suit, mama. Even—and maybe especially—if you have stretch marks.

Personally, I've never had a flat stomach a day in my life, and I never felt more confident and comfortable in a bathing suit than I did when I was pregnant. Who needs a flat stomach when you have a baby bump? No sucking in or flexing required to look cute. Let it all hang out. This is a great practice in loving yourself and your changing body and embracing the physical changes motherhood brings.

If you're headed to the beach for your babymoon or chilling poolside close to home, don't forget to apply lots of sunscreen to your bump and the rest of your body. Pregnancy makes you more susceptible to sunburn.

Ready to do it? Here are tips for finding a good maternity swimsuit:

- If you're self-conscious about stretch marks, look for high-waisted bottoms. These are also great for wearing after you have the baby, as your body shrinks back down.
- Find stores that let you buy bottoms and tops separately. You may need a bigger size for one of the pieces.
- Maternity suits aren't always necessary. You can make low-cut bottoms and bikini tops work. Try pairing a maternity tankini top with regular bottoms, or maternity bottoms with a bikini top.
- Lightly padded tops will work best to absorb breast milk and colostrum leaks before and after baby is born.

If it's the dead of winter, forget the bikini and lounge in your undies, or wear special lingerie. Try to release your insecurities and focus all your love and attention on your glorious belly. You made that! Be proud.

YOUR BODY RIGHT NOW

Tiffany Reese, stylist and body positivity blogger at Lookie Boo

Focus on how powerful and magical your body has become. That's what really helped me. Your body is a vessel that is creating human life. I know that my body and life will never be the same, and thank God, because this new life with my babies is so much better than I ever could ever have ever imagined! And remember that this body shape is temporary.

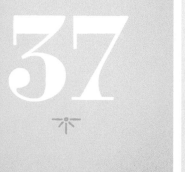

SET UP A NOTIFICATION PLAN

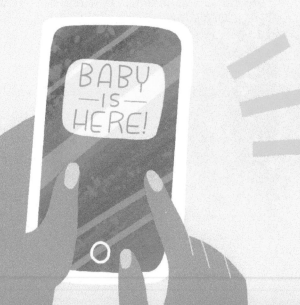

HAVEN'T YOU HAD YOUR BABY YET???
What about now? Now? Are you having contractions now?

You may want to throw things at people who insist on asking you, "When are you going to have that baby?" If so, congratulations! You are normal.

Eventually, you will have to tell people when the baby arrives, though. Putting a plan in place now will not only make it easier for you to spread the word later, it will also ease loved ones' minds that they will not miss out on the news when it's time. They're on the A-list—no risk of learning about it from your Insta feed. These are some things to think about.

When labor begins. Are you planning to post to social media, text, or call people when you go into labor, or will you have someone do some texting and calling for you? Or would you rather keep it private and just show up when you have a picture of a baby to share? Letting people know you're experiencing contractions can be fun, but it can also ramp up the texting and the tagging and the calling to check on you.

When things get real. Determine who is going to be in charge of fielding calls and texts when go time is here. I recommend either handing your phone over to your partner or labor support person, or turning it off once you're in active labor or head into the operating room if you have a C-section.

Consider how those closest to you would best receive the news. Sure, your coworkers and distant relatives can find out when you post about it to your Facebook page. But your immediate family and best friends would likely love a group text and a few pictures first, and your grandma probably wants to find out via a phone call.

When the baby's here. Put your mom, partner, or someone else close to you in charge of making phone calls once baby arrives. Have a list of people you want to text right away, and plan to pass those off to your partner. Then let everyone know how they will find out.

"Don't worry! You'll know as soon as it happens because my mom is going to call you. Until then, no news is, well, no news."
While you're at it, be sure to ask your friends and family to wait for you to share the news on social media first. Well-meaning loved ones may be excited to post pictures and tag you before you've had a chance to make your child's birth Facebook-official. Which is annoying at best.

If after all this, you still have people asking if you've had your baby yet, feel free to direct them to HaveYouHadThatBabyYet.com.

38

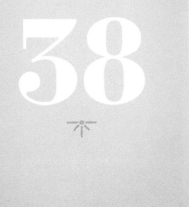

PACK YOUR BAGS

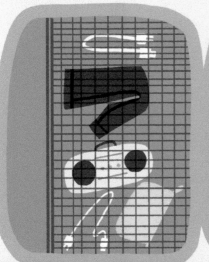
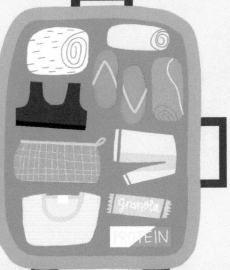

*T*his is just like a vacay! Except you'll be coming home wearing mesh undies and accompanied by a stowaway much cuter than a bedbug. Time to pack your bags for your breezy trip to labor and delivery!

There are at least two people you need to pack for if you're birthing away from home: yourself and your baby. But you may also want to bring some things for your partner, too.

Mama's bag checklist:

Small extension cord. This is so helpful when your bed is in the middle of the room with the outlet 10 feet away, and you want to charge your phone and use it at the same time.

Portable bluetooth speaker or radio. Your hospital may offer something like this already, so check with them before you pack it.

Comfy bra to labor in. Any color is fine, unless you plan to be in the water. Then, a black sports bra is perfect, especially if you plan to have pictures taken while you labor.

Warm socks or slippers with grip. The hospital will provide you with some nonskid options, but you can always pack some of your own.

Flip-flops. For showering or laboring in and out of water.

Labor tools, like tennis balls or a heating pad. Check with your hospital, as they may already have things like this there. I once rolled up to the hospital with my own yoga ball when it was unnecessary.

Snacks. I like to pack a bag with chocolate, Jell-O, pudding, pretzels, and sports drinks in a small cooler.

Toiletries. Anything you'd pack for an overnight stay elsewhere. I'd also bring a hair tie, lip balm, and facial wipes.

Your own soft towel. The hospital towels can be small and stiff.

Comfy clothes. Black or dark-colored lounge pants or pajamas will keep you from feeling self-conscious about postpartum bleeding. Bring some soft, stretchy nursing bras, too. A robe might make you feel a little more "dressed" if you have visitors (like your in-laws) whom you don't want to see you in your PJs.

A coming-home outfit for yourself. Pull something from your maternity wardrobe. It's not uncommon to gain 40 pounds and lose 15 during childbirth. You get the gist—the old clothes are a ways off.

A breastfeeding pillow or pillow you can't sleep without. Hospitals have pillows, of course, but they aren't very firm or fluffy, in my experience. Breastfeeding pillows can really help when you're trying to position a newborn. If you need a special pillow to sleep, definitely bring that, too.

Of course, once this bag is packed, put a note on top of it with a reminder to grab your packed snack cooler and a list of the things you need to add to it before you head out the door. For example: cell phone, wallet, insurance card, camera, toothbrush, makeup, and any chargers you need for electronics.

Diaper bag checklist:

Baby lotion. Some hospitals don't provide this, and I've always found my babies get really dry skin.

Pacifiers. I'll just say that, in my opinion, pacifiers can be great, even from day one. It's never harmed my breastfeeding relationships. If you feel differently, cool, don't worry about them. But if you think you may want one, pack a couple of different brands in newborn sizes.

Baby clothes, hats, and blankets. The hospital will provide these, but if you want to dress your baby and swaddle them in those cute outfits you washed and folded, you can. You'll want something for them to wear home, for sure, and you can always add a blanket to the car seat if it's cold out.

For your partner:

Check with your hospital to see if they provide a foldout couch and any blankets or pillows for partners. Some won't even have a chair for them to sleep in; others may feel like a hotel for both of you. You won't know unless you ask.

YOU DO YOU

There is no right amount of stuff to bring with you. If you're good with using the hospital's pillows and towels, that's great! And if you "over-pack," I promise you won't be the first or last parent who does. Overall, there's no one right way to do parenting, right down to what you pack to have a baby. You just have to do you. Casey Brown, transgender parent and blogger at *Life with Roozle*, puts it pretty powerfully:

"With everything we do, it's because of who we are, our personality. But being pregnant? Somehow that becomes some kind of universal experience where everyone somehow has the right to tell you how to do it. I'm a researcher by nature. When pregnant with my first baby, people told me I was bananas for researching everything, for creating a spreadsheet of the registry, and using apps for feeding schedules. But to me, given my personality, this wasn't about being a scared first-time parent, it was about pregnancy being a project. And I love projects. If your personality is to roll with it, allow yourself to roll with pregnancy. If your personality is to freak out, go ahead and freak out about preg-nancy, too."

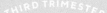

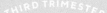THIRD TRIMESTER

39

PICK OUT BIRTH ANNOUNCEMENTS

Introducing: Samuel James

8 lbs 12oz + 21 in.

On a scale of 1 to HOLY COW, I'M ABOUT TO HAVE A BABY, this is pretty high up there. It's time to envision, budget, and plan for how you want to officially announce to your loved ones that you've had a baby.

But wait, didn't I just tell you how to tell them all via text and social media? Right, yes. Most people are already going to know you had a baby before they get your announcement because we live in a world of high-speed digital communication, but this a more formal way to introduce your baby to your friends and family and show off a photo or two. It also makes a nice keepsake for your baby's memory box and your grandma's refrigerator.

Figure out what your budget will allow for this before you decide which option is best. (And if your budget is zero, keep reading, I've got a tip for you at the end of this.) If you're planning to mail paper announcements, make a list of the people you'd like to send them to so you can get an idea of how many you need to order. Don't forget to include stamps in your total estimated cost.

Also, now is a really great time to create a good system for storing addresses. Some online card services allow you to keep an address book with them, and they'll even address the envelopes for you! I enthusiastically recommend that option, but if you don't go that route, try to enter addresses into a program on your computer that will make it easy to print your own envelopes. A great time to start gathering and entering these addresses is when you write out thank-you cards after your baby shower, if you have one.

If you want to go with announcements with photos and/or details printed on them, the announcements will have to wait to be ordered for obvious reasons, but you can still narrow down your favorites and start looking for discount codes and coupons that won't expire before you're able to order them.

Are you planning to have the photo printed directly on the announcement, or will you include a separate print? Be sure to budget for the cost of photo prints if you're going with a separate print. Some families opt to use professional photos from a newborn or family photo session. If you don't plan to do this, think of how you'll get the photos you want to use. Will you be taking them yourself? It doesn't hurt to practice with something like a teddy bear, using the same lighting and camera that you plan to use to photograph your baby.

Timing is pretty loose when it comes to when you should send these. You're not obligated to send them to anyone at a certain time, so don't stress yourself out. There's no need to be stuffing envelopes five weeks postpartum unless you want to, but it could be worth adjusting your time frame to combine your baby announcement with, for example, a holiday or New Year's card.

If you can't or don't want to spend money on paper announcements, there are beautiful online announcements that are free! Paperless Post offers e-card options that are just as gorgeous as high-end card designs (and you can often print a few as keepsakes for a small fee), and graphic design software Canva will let you custom-make one using one of its templates.

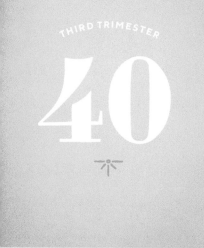

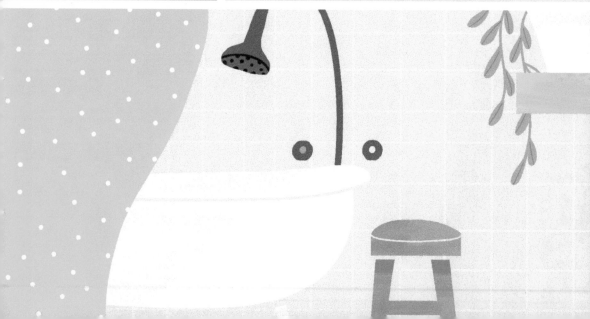

THIRD TRIMESTER

40

ALLOW
YOURSELF TO
BE MISERABLE
AND WHINE

*L*isten, it's totally normal right now to be OVER being pregnant. People love to tell moms at this stage that "baby will come when they are ready," and yes, friend, it's okay to find that condescending and to stab them with your eyes. It is also okay to dream of putting a hex on anyone who tells you to enjoy sleep while you can right now. Like you're even *able* to sleep?!

You're a logical grown-up, so obviously you understand how calendars work and you know that it's just a waiting game right now. That does not mean you have to like waiting. That doesn't even mean you can't cry about waiting. That's right, girl. You go have a seat in your shower—literally bring a chair in there if you need to because standing is hard right now—and have yourself a good cry. Or lock yourself in your room with the lights off and the TV on, and give yourself permission to not answer texts or talk to anyone while you pout about still being pregnant.

Speaking of texts and calls, notify your people that you're not taking any if they are asking if you're still pregnant. Tell them they can contact your partner with questions, or they can just mind their own business and wait for your announcement in your own time.

I do advise trying not to dwell on feeling like you'll be pregnant forever for too long. After you've had your cry and pout fest, distract yourself by doing anything that makes you happy. Treat yourself to a coffee, ask your partner to rub your feet, window-shop at your favorite store.

This is actually another great opportunity to prioritize your self-care as a parent. Let yourself feel what you're feeling. Set boundaries with other people. Then take care of yourself in the best way you know how. Also, don't be afraid to reach out and ask for help or companionship. A dinner with a friend who vows not to inquire about your cervix's nonexistent dilation can do wonders for the weary pregnant-forever soul.

And take pictures of those swollen feet and that larger-than-life belly! Don't stop documenting your pregnancy just because you hate life right now. One of my most cherished pictures of my last pregnancy is of my hilariously large, bare belly taken while I hibernated in our bed. I do not look happy in the picture. I wasn't. But now, it's amazing to look back on that moment. I'm also saving it to show my son anytime he claims I don't love him. LOOK WHAT MY BODY DID FOR YOU.

41

PLAN GIFTS OF GRATITUDE

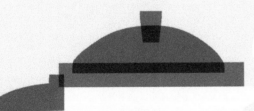
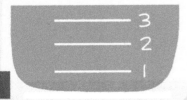
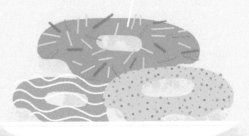

thank you ♡

$\mathcal{E}$**very time I had a baby, my midwives, the** nurses, and certified nurse assistants who helped me through it were like angels on earth. I have so much love in my heart for each of them to this day. I hope you get just as lucky and that the person who helps you walk to the bathroom for the first time after giving birth treats you with as much kindness and dignity as each of mine have. I hope they do kind things for you like show you how to make icicle pads for your mesh panties or hold you up while you shower.

Whether they are your nurses, doctor, midwife, or doula, these medical and care providers can quickly become people you feel immensely thankful for. While you are counting down the days to baby's arrival, take some time to plan out how you can express your gratitude toward them for holding your leg while you pushed and casually cleaning up *everything* you pushed out, or for helping you focus and remain calm while your OB made your C-section incision.

There's no need to get super elaborate or spend a lot of money. A simple thank-you card can go a long way. Pack a stack of blank cards and a nice pen in your hospital bag. You'll be able to fill out cards for nurses while you're there and drop them off at the central desk on your way out.

If you want to do something after the fact, I definitely recommend at least writing down or making a note in your phone of the nurses' names and one or two specific things they did that you can thank them for.

Beyond a handwritten note, some other nice ways to show your appreciation:

Coffee delivery. Send your partner out to pick up a coffee order for your nurses while you're recovering, or come back in a few weeks with a box of hot coffee and maybe some doughnuts for the L&D staff on duty that day to share.

Pizza. Order pizza for everyone working that night!

Gift cards. If there's a drive-through nearby or a coffee shop in the hospital, pick up some gift cards and include them in your thank-you cards.

A letter of praise to their supervisor. If a nurse or caregiver has gone above and beyond to make you feel taken care of, write a letter to their supervisor and sing their praises.

SAYING THANKS

LaShawn Wiltz, RN and labor and delivery nurse

I've received everything from money to food to flowers, but once a family gave me a gift certificate for a massage because I pushed with that poor girl for three hours, begging her doctor for just a little more time. She delivered vaginally and the whole family was happy. It was so sweet.

LOVE, BACKATCHA

If you've been fortunate to have a supportive partner beside you through all this, you've probably experienced a spectrum of emotions for them, from anger that they brought you home a cheeseburger with mustard on it, to deep love for all the times they rubbed your feet and didn't question your need for a 65-degree house. Without a doubt, this has been as big a life change for them as you.

Think of some ways you can celebrate this new adventure with your partner. You don't have to wait for Father's or Mother's Day to gift them a cheesy coffee mug with a picture of your baby on it. And a heartfelt note about how much their support has meant to you is a lovely token of gratitude any day of the year.

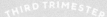THIRD TRIMESTER

42

HAVE A REAL TALK AND RELAX DAY WITH YOUR BESTIES

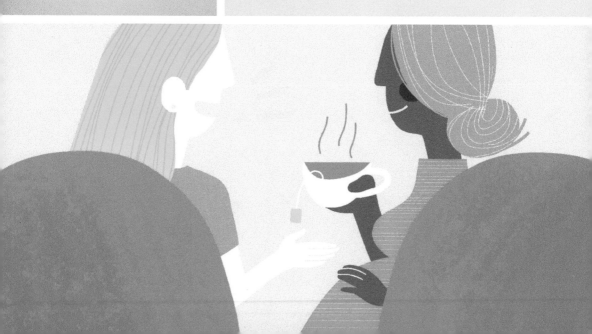

When the general public asks how you're feeling, you probably respond with "fine" or maybe "a little tired but good," even though you want to shout, "I HAVEN'T SLEPT IN SIX WEEKS AND I WOKE UP CHOKING ON MY OWN STOMACH ACID LAST NIGHT, BUT I'M SWELL, THANKS FOR ASKING."

It's just not worth the energy to get real with most people. And goodness knows if you do, you set yourself up for them to reply, "Be grateful! You're so blessed! Enjoy these moments." (Side note: You can be grateful and also hate these moments at the same time.)

But your best friends? THEY will listen respectfully to the real answer to "How are you feeling?" And if they've been through pregnancy before, they'll be eager to commiserate. Be intentional about connecting with your friends right now. You may or may not have had a baby shower, but this date is all about you being with the people you are closest with. No games, no presents.

Invite your besties over for brunch or tea and cookies. I love the idea of making it a PJs party, because that means you don't have to get out of your stretchy pants. But if the idea of slipping on a dress right now perks you up, then go for it. The key is to make it comfortable for YOU. Your friends will understand and be game for whatever you decide.

Then lay it all out there. Be honest, be vulnerable, be real. Tell them what you're scared of. Tell them what you can't wait for. If they are parents, ask them if they ever pooped while pushing. Ask them if sex was different after baby. Ask them how it felt the first night they were home with their newborn and what their go-to trick is for getting a fussy baby to sleep.

This can feel like an anxious and uncertain time. You're so close to becoming a mom, but there's still so much you feel like you don't know. Even if your friends don't have babies of their own and can't give you any good answers, just having someone who will listen to you and withhold judgment is priceless.

If you can't make a day of it—maybe your BFF lives three states away—chat on the phone or via Skype. Whatever you do, don't shut your friends out now. Don't keep your worries and wonders to yourself.

FRIENDS WITHOUT KIDS

Lindsay Murphy Maloan, mother of three

While my friends had no idea what I was experiencing, they were quick to provide support and help in whatever way I needed it. Paint the nursery in exchange for beer and pizza? Sure! Help me put on a garage sale while my husband is out of town? Absolutely! They were never too busy or too tired to be our support system. I returned the favor by being their designated driver several times. My son became their baby, too; an only child to 12 really awesome friend parents, who to this day are still our core group of friends whom we refer to as our "framily." I often feel bad that I haven't been able to return all of the favors to them during their pregnancies, because I'm now chasing three kids of my own.

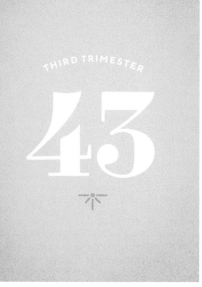

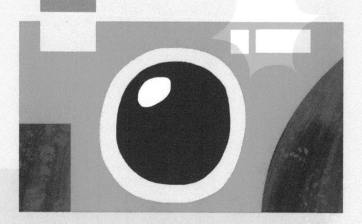

THIRD TRIMESTER

43

MAKE A PLAN FOR PICTURES AND VIDEO

IN THE DELIVERY ROOM

Your baby's birth is one of those moments that you'll never get back. There are no makeups or second chances for pictures of their first minutes earthside. So it's well worth putting a little thought into how you want to document this.

Professional birth photographers are increasingly common, so if you'd like to delegate the task of capturing your baby's entrance into the world, you shouldn't have a problem finding someone with the skills and equipment to do so. Before you hire the first person you find on Google, though, be sure to meet with them. This is someone who will be with you for one of the most intimate and special moments of your life. It's very important that you feel comfortable with them and that you feel confident they will support your labor choices and respect your care providers.

If you'll be counting on your partner to take photos and/or video, establish some ground rules early on and give them some guidance for what you want. Once you're in active labor, you're probably not going to feel like directing things. You may even completely forget about cameras.

Go over when and where you want pictures and video taken. Are crowning shots off-limits or something you want them to be sure to capture? Make your wishes and expectations clear. Also, if you're delivering outside of the home, especially in a hospital, check what the policy is for cameras in the room, and note that the policy may be different if you're delivering via C-section.

BIRTH PHOTOGRAPHY TIPS

Katie Lacer, birth photographer, MommaKTShoots.com

1. **GET TO KNOW YOUR CAMERA PRIOR TO THE BIG DAY.** Knowing how to do simple things, like turning a flash on and off or changing basic settings, can make a huge difference not only in your comfort level but also in your ability to actually document your baby's arrival.

2. **USE YOUR LIGHT!** Open blinds or curtains when you can, and capitalize on light coming from an open door or even a computer monitor. Don't be afraid of dim or dark birth spaces, either; you can often move around for beautiful shadows without needing to use a flash.

3. **MOVE AROUND AND GET SOME VARIETY.** It's easy to get stuck in one spot. Low angles are great for wide-angle or full-room shots; straight-on is great for details; and above is wonderful for faces and bodies. Hop up on a chair or stool for a bird's-eye view.

4. **DOCUMENT THE DETAILS.** Those little things, like the clock showing the time of day, the room number, or the midwife's kit, will help fill out your baby's story.

5. **PREPARE FOR THE RUSH.** At some point things are going to speed up. Most of the time, staying near Mom's shoulder will give you the most bang for your buck as far as being able to get baby coming earthside (no matter how the baby is born!) along with Mom's expression. When applicable, follow the baby!

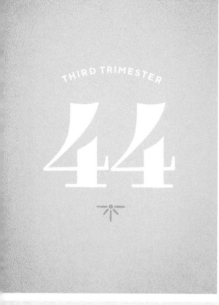

MAKE A FEEDING PLAN

BREAST, BOTTLE, OR BOTH?

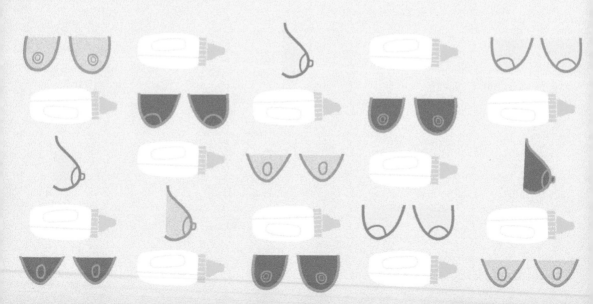

I really wish feeding babies was as simple as deciding you're going to breastfeed or bottle-feed, and then just doing that. But the truth is, no matter how you want to feed your baby, there's some education and preparation involved.

If you plan to breastfeed, it's really important to learn how and when your body makes breast milk. It doesn't just happen; there's a little learning curve. You have to put your baby on your breasts to signal your body to make milk, and for best results it's important to do this frequently and as early as possible. Ask your provider now if they will help you get skin-to-skin contact with your baby immediately after baby is born and let your baby try to nurse soon after that. Skin-to-skin contact after birth has a variety of benefits, including helping your baby regulate their body temperature and making them more likely to "latch on" for breastfeeding. Depending on your hospital, you may be able to do this even if you have a C-section, but definitely communicate that this is something you want to happen.

You can learn a lot about breastfeeding before you have your baby by reading breastfeeding books and talking with your friends and relatives who have breastfed, but nothing teaches you like actually having a baby to feed. Read up before baby gets here, but also be ready and open to do some learning after they arrive. Your hospital or birthing center will probably have a lactation consultant (LC) on staff, and she's a valuable person to meet with before you go home.

Additionally, get contact information for an LC or breastfeeding support group you can visit, or who can come visit you, if you have any problems later on.

While there is a lot of pressure on moms to try to breastfeed, some moms simply can't or don't want to—and that's fine! There's still, however, a bit of preparation that also goes into planning to bottle-feed formula to your baby.

First, check with your hospital to see if they provide formula for you to feed your baby or if you need to bring your own. You may want to use a brand other than what they're offering, so be prepared to pack and bring that if needed. Some babies can even be picky about what type of bottle they like best. I recommend having one each of a few different brands, seeing which one works best for you and baby, and then investing in more after you've established a winner.

Baby-Feeding Tips from Jocelyn Slaughter, MD:

1. If you decide to breastfeed, make sure your partner is aware and understands that they will still have to participate and help in the process.

2. Understand that it can be a frustrating process; however, there are many resources that the hospital has, and there are postpartum breastfeeding support groups, to assist you.

3. The whole point is to feed your baby. If your baby is not getting enough from breastfeeding, your pediatrician may recommend supplementing with formula when all other recommendations have still not increased your baby's weight. Do not look at yourself as a failure—as long as you are providing nutrients for your baby, through the breasts or not, you are a winner and a great mom.

OWN YOUR DECISIONS

Lizz Porter, mom of one and blogger at More Than Thursdays

As a kidney transplant recipient, breastfeeding was never an option for me. I knew I'd use formula from the day I found out I was pregnant. For a new mom, I'd just really encourage her to be comfortable with and confident in her decision. It can be hard in this heavy "breast is best" world to be a formula-feeding mom, but whatever it takes to make sure your baby is healthy is what matters.

ROLL WITH THE DETOURS

It's okay if this whole baby-feeding plan goes out the window. It is wonderful to be totally committed to breastfeeding your baby. Personally, I had to work very hard at it the first time around, and I'm glad I stuck with it. But I know many moms who worked even harder, and it ultimately wasn't worth the toll it was taking on their mental health. Parenting is a life lesson in learning to go with what works. Don't feel guilty if your best-laid plans end up changing.

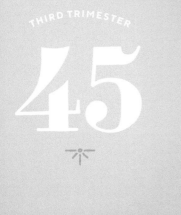

45

STOCK FEEDING SUPPLIES

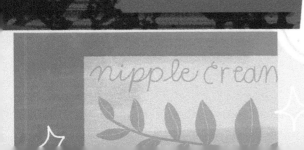

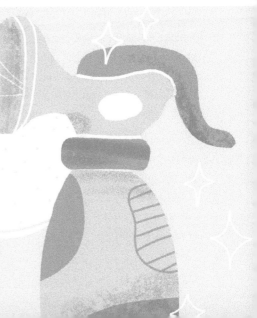

*N*ow that you've given some thought to how you hope to feed your baby, you'll want to take a little time to gather supplies that will help you succeed.

If you plan to breastfeed:

Nipple cream. Your hospital may provide this for you, but if you have a specific brand you love, it's worth packing your own.

Breast pads. You won't need these until your milk comes in, and that probably won't be until you're home. Once it does come in, however, you can go through a lot of them while your supply evens out. But if you don't, don't worry—milk leakage is not an indicator of a good supply.

Manual pump. At first that might not make sense to you, because maybe you're planning to exclusively breastfeed, especially in the beginning. Why would you need a pump? Well, even if you never plan to give your baby a bottle, I highly recommend getting a manual pump, because it helps with engorgement (breasts overfilling) in the beginning, and it's very handy for travel later on.

Electric pump. This is not necessarily a must-have. If you are planning to be away from your baby for only a few hours every now and then, your manual pump will probably be all you need. If you will go back to a job out of the home and away from your baby, though, definitely look into a good-quality double-electric pump, which may be covered by insurance.

Bottles and milk storage. Again, even if you don't think you'll bottle-feed your baby, it's still good to have these things on hand just in case you have to go somewhere unexpectedly or your partner wants a turn at feeding the baby.

If you plan to formula-feed:

Formula. Ask your pediatrician's advice on what brand will likely work best for your baby. You may need to change this up, so don't stockpile too much of one type in the beginning.

Bottles. Just like with breastfeeding, you'll never know what baby is going to love, so don't invest too much in just one brand in the beginning.

Formula dispenser. If you use a powdered formula, you'll need a way to portion it out into individual bottle amounts, especially when you're out of the house. There are bottles and dispensers on the market that do this for you, or you can use preportioned packets of powder.

Bottle-sterilizing system. This could be a stand-alone bottle sterilizer that sits on your counter, microwaveable bags meant for pump parts, or simply your dishwasher or a pot of boiling water.

FORMULA TIPS

Suzanne Barston, author of Bottled Up *and blogger at* Fearless Formula Feeder

"The best advice I can give for parents with a newborn who know they want to bottle-feed is to use ready-to-feed (RTF) formula for the first few weeks. There's far less chance of human error, which is a good thing when you're a new parent going on two hours of sleep. Using RTF is safer, although more expensive; you don't need to worry about the water you're mixing it with, and if you use the disposable nursers (the ones that come in 2- to 4-ounce sizes) there's no need to sterilize bottles. You can switch to the cheaper powder after a few weeks, but for those crazy first days, RTF formula is your best friend.

For those who have just given birth: A snug (but not too tight) sports bra, some cold cabbage, ibuprofen, and Sudafed. You'll be glad to have these things to keep yourself comfy when your milk is drying up. Put the cold cabbage leaves in your bra to cover your breasts for some soothing relief. The ibuprofen will help with the pain, and the Sudafed helps dry up your milk supply.

BREASTFEEDING FIRST AID

As mentioned, there can be a learning curve to breastfeeding your baby, and while you and your body try to sort things out, there can be some discomfort. My faves are the booby tubes from Earth Mama Organics. One bonus is that these aren't a single-use purchase: they'll double as boo-boo soothers when your child gets big enough to scrape their knee.

When I experienced engorgement, I had a hard time getting my newborns to latch on, so I had to express some milk first. This is when my manual pump did the most work for me. I liked to stand in a hot shower and pump with my handheld manual pump straight into a bottle until the breast softened enough to get the baby to latch on. After my shower, I would nurse the baby, then apply a generous amount of nipple cream and place the warm cloth tubes inside my bra.

If you are experiencing extreme discomfort and pain while breastfeeding, reach out to a lactation consultant or a breastfeeding support group.

46

CREATE A POSTPARTUM MENTAL HEALTH PLAN

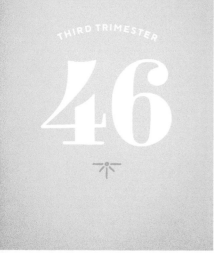

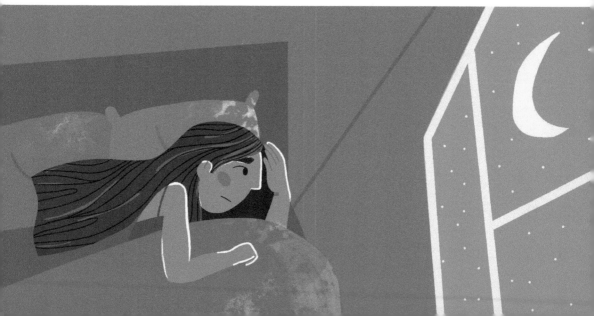

*J*ust like you would have a safety net of people you can talk to and a backup plan in place if you have issues feeding your baby, you should also have a safety net in place in case you experience a postpartum mood and anxiety disorder. Perinatal mood and anxiety disorders affect at least one in seven mothers, and if you are a woman of color, you are unfortunately at even greater risk.

Most of us picture a mom who can't stop crying and whose baby is a newborn when we think of someone with postpartum depression, and that can be the case. But it can also set in up to a year post-birth, long after the six week postpartum checkup when many of our providers check in with us for the last time. And most people don't even realize that postpartum anxiety, obsessive-compulsive disorder (OCD), or psychosis (which occurs in only 0.1 to 0.2 percent of births) exist.

I experienced postpartum anxiety and OCD (in the form of intrusive thoughts) after all four of my babies, but it took me until I felt like I was suffering from a heart attack when my second baby was nine months old before I got help. It never occurred to me that I was sick. I didn't feel depressed. I didn't cry. Instead, I felt intense rage and couldn't stop thinking of all the ways everyone I knew would die. I couldn't walk near stairs without vividly imagining accidentally throwing my baby off them.

It is my sincere hope that you will not feel alarmed by this, because postpartum mood and anxiety disorders are absolutely treatable. But it is so important to know what to look for, so tell your partner and your loved ones what to look for, and have a plan in place in case you or the people around you begin to suspect that you are experiencing postpartum mental health challenges.

Symptoms to look out for:

- Feelings of overwhelm and hopelessness
- Feelings of sadness or emptiness
- Guilt
- Panic
- Racing thoughts
- Inability to relax
- Sleeping a lot or not much at all
- Loss of appetite
- Loss of focus

- Anger
- Fear
- Disturbing thoughts
- Intense desire to keep checking on things or on your baby
- Unprovoked inability to trust those around you

If you begin to feel any of these symptoms, the first thing you should do is reach out to your OB, midwife, or family doctor, no matter how old your baby is. You can discuss treatment options with them, like medication and therapy. They may want to run blood work or other tests as well.

Next, find a psychotherapist who is trained in treating perinatal mood disorders. Your provider may have one they recommend; otherwise, call the Postpartum Support International Warmline at 1-800-944-4773, and they'll connect you with a local coordinator who can get you in touch with a therapist or support group.

Keep these resources accessible, and share them with your partner and close family. Maintain an open and proactive dialogue with your provider and loved ones, encouraging them to help you look out for any symptoms. If you are the one in seven who has a mood disorder, you'll be ready.

DEALING WITH THE HARD STUFF

Elaine H. Cavazos, LCSW

You are your best and most powerful advocate. Having a baby is a transformational experience, and with it comes joy, love, and happiness, as well as pain, sadness, and sometimes regret. It's okay to talk about the hard stuff and the hard feelings. Find a space, whether it's in individual therapy, a support or therapy group, and/or with trusted friends and loved ones, where you can be real about your feelings and how you are doing as you take on what is arguably the most important work of your life. Know that though you may feel very alone, you are not, and there are people out there who really want to be that kind and supportive ear. And finally, maybe most importantly, you are the most important person in your baby's life. They love you powerfully and they don't expect perfection. Lean into that love, and know that it is always okay to ask for help.

47

PREPARE FOR PUMPING

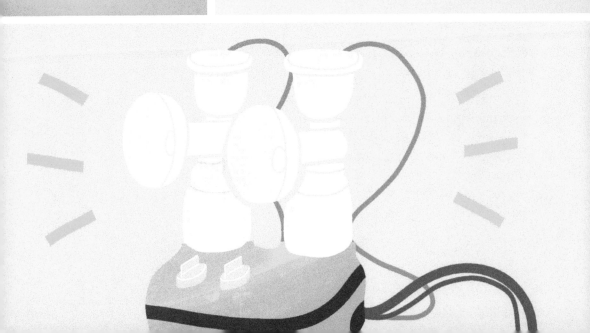

*I*f you plan to breastfeed, even for a short amount of time, there's a good chance you'll have to pump or express breast milk at some point. If you're bottle-feeding, skip on down to the next to-do.

For some moms, pumping is not something they have to do regularly, but for others, it's the sole source of food for their babies. Either way, there's a good chance you'll become accustomed to the whoosh-whoosh of a milking machine soon.

Jessica Martin-Webber, mom of seven and blogger at *The Leaky Boob*, has this sage wisdom for prospective pumping parents:

Lube it up and, yes, size matters. If you plan on pumping, buy breast pump flanges in a couple of sizes in your third trimester (breasts change during pregnancy) so you will have the correct size postpartum. Flanges that are too big or small can result in tissue damage, low milk supply, and pain. Pain can also happen with friction, so rub those flanges with some safe nipple cream.

Get it covered. Your pump may be free through your insurance, so check with a DME (durable medical equipment supply company) to see what is covered.

Better isn't always better. Determine your pumping lifestyle needs before getting your pump. You may not need to pump at all if you're not planning on being away from your baby, or you may need to pump 12 times a day if you are exclusively pumping. Figure out what your needs will be and select a pump that fits those needs. No need for a high-power double-electric fancy pump if you're only going to pump for an occasional Friday-evening date—a hand pump will do.

Get handy and don't watch. Hands-on breast massage while pumping can help increase output to the pump and loosen the fat globules that stick on the insides of your milk ducts, which is important in fully emptying the breasts so your body gets the signal to make more milk, protecting your milk supply. A hands-free pumping bra goes a long way in helping with this. As you massage, don't watch your pumping output; focus on something else (such as a video of your baby). It will go faster, and you'll be more relaxed, optimizing output.

Be flexible. It takes time and practice to work out breastfeeding and pumping. Be patient and be prepared to be flexible. Commit to feeding your baby first, putting methodology second. The first rule of lactation support is "feed the baby," and the second rule is "protect supply." Your friends may have had one experience and loved a certain breast pump, but your journey belongs to you and your baby, and may look different. Having flexible expectations can help you adapt easily along the way.

48

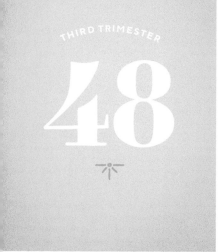

LET PEOPLE KNOW WHEN THEY CAN VISIT

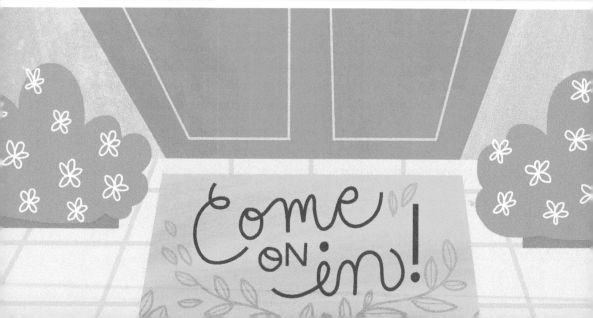

*N*ow is a great time to think about who you want, and who will be allowed, to visit you right after you give birth, and to make sure well-meaning family and friends know when and where their presence is requested. So much of parenting is putting up boundaries, and it starts from day one.

If you plan to give birth in a hospital, check into their visitor policy and hours. Some will not allow children who are not siblings to visit. Many have specific visiting hours. All hospitals request that anyone with a cold stay home.

If you have a home birth or will be back home for recovery after delivering at a birth center, it's good to establish your own visitor policies for the house.

Those first few hours and days are so important for bonding with your baby and, if you choose to breastfeed, laying the groundwork for a successful breastfeeding relationship. Too many visitors for too long can get in the way of all that.

After the baby is born, I recommend sending a text or message stating what time visitors can stop by, and including the time they need to leave. Have someone else send this, like your partner or other support person, and give them strict instructions to adhere to it and not to notify you if anyone is giving them any pushback about it. They are your bouncer after baby is born.

"Hey, Aunt Margaret! The baby is here! He's a handsome little guy, born at 6:35 this morning. (Your name here) will be up for visitors today from 3 to 4. Please tell Sally we would love to see her and the kids, if they're all healthy, in two weeks at our house!"

Also, come up with a phrase or a word you can say that will signal your bouncer to encourage a visitor to get moving.

There will be plenty of time for people to meet and hold your new baby. It's so important that you make your recovery and bonding with the baby the number-one focus immediately after they are born. Come up with a plan now so you don't get stuck in an awkward situation after baby arrives.

VISITING RULES

Stephanie Precourt, mother of three

Setting boundaries and expectations for family and friends before baby arrives will help prevent hurt feelings from well-meaning loved ones, and it is a necessary act of care for your postpartum self. Just because you're giving birth at home doesn't mean your "home" will operate as usual. I had friends who were open to their entire family being present during and after birth—they made it a party. I personally needed quiet solitude and was thankful that I had set visiting hours for family and friends, including grandparents. Gifts and meals can be left on the doorstep for the first few days, and I don't recall anyone being offended about that.

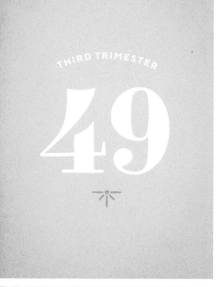

THIRD TRIMESTER

49

GET SOME
SLEEP, OR AT
LEAST TRY

*B*etween the back and hip pain, the reflux, the insomnia, the constantly pressed bladder, and how hard it can be to breathe with a foot in your ribs, sleep is not necessarily a thing that comes easy in the third trimester. And yet? You are desperately wanting to sleep, is my guess.

Okay, let's talk about some ways we can try to make that happen for you.

Back and hip pain. Make yourself a nest of pillows—a FORTRESS of pillows if you need to, although sometimes it takes only a well-placed pillow behind your back, and sometimes many little pillows works better than one giant, expensive pregnancy pillow. Topical pain relief, like a muscle cream or essential oils, can also help long enough to enable you to doze off.

Reflux. If you've woken up choking on your own vomit while pregnant, you are not alone. Welcome to a really lousy club. Sleeping slightly inclined, either propped up on pillows or lying back in a recliner, can help if you can find a comfortable side-lying position.

There are also a few acid reflux medications that are safe to take while pregnant, and these can help tremendously. Of course, check with your medical provider first. Also, avoid heavy or greasy meals a few hours before bedtime.

Insomnia. This can be caused by many things, but if you feel like you can't turn your brain off, try emptying it out. Write down your thoughts or fears or whatever else is keeping you up in a journal. Sometimes it helps to just get up and do something instead of lying in bed tossing and turning and getting mad that you're not sleeping. Try a meditation app on your phone to help focus on deep breathing and relaxation.

Your overworked bladder. The best way to decrease the number of times you need to pee at night is to gradually decrease your fluid intake in the evening and fully empty your bladder before bed. Now, this means you need to be sure you're getting plenty of water throughout the rest of the day. And if you're thirsty at 9:00 p.m., drink something, okay? Don't stop hydrating, just cut back. When you use the restroom before bed, try leaning side to side and all the way forward to see if you can literally squeeze every last drop of pee out.

Trouble breathing. Unfortunately, as real estate in your abdomen becomes scarce, it can become hard to take a deep breath. First, you want to ensure that nothing serious is keeping you from fully inhaling, so be sure your medical provider is in the know. If it appears that you're just the victim of a giant baby doing a fully extended handstand on your hips, it could be worth visiting a chiropractor who specializes in dealing with pregnant women. Speaking from personal experience, I found out why I had been so winded when my chiro discovered that my angelic baby had separated two of my ribs and kicked another out of place. He was able to put everything back where it went painlessly. I can't even describe how life changing that was.

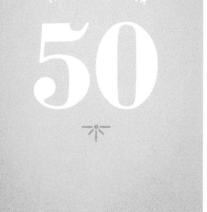

THIRD TRIMESTER

50

PLAN BABY'S FIRST FASHION STATEMENT

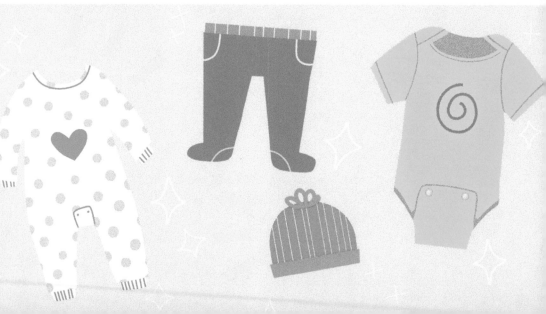

*T*his is so fun. I'm so excited for you! You've made it through many medical appointments, had your blood drawn so much you know which vein is your "good" one, and now you get to envision what tiny ensemble you'll put baby in when you leave the hospital or birth center, or when you welcome baby's first guests to your home.

Go all in! Let yourself enjoy this. Your baby's clothes will never be cuter, and you will never love doing laundry more than when their onesies are the size of a kitten.

It is a little challenging dressing someone you've never seen or met before. Here are a few tips for picking out baby's first important outfits:

Get two sizes! It's really hard to predict how big a baby will be before they are born. Estimates based on ultrasounds can be off by up to two pounds in either direction. Those two pounds can be the difference between squeezing your roly-poly into a newborn romper or having to size up to a 0 to 3 months outfit. If you know you'll be delivering your baby early, it's smart to find a few things in preemie size.

Dress baby for indoor temperatures. No need to buy your newborn a teeny parka for the ride home from the hospital. Chances are, they're going to go straight from the hospital lobby into your car under the covered valet station. A blanket and a hat, in addition to a lightweight full-coverage outfit, are all you'll need to keep them warm. Conversely, bringing a summer baby home in nothing but a T-shirt could make them uncomfortable if the AC is blasting during the ride.

Have a backup. Newborn poop can be explosive. One minute you're buckling baby into their seat, waiting for your hospital discharge papers, the next you're peeling a yellow-poop-drenched sleeper off your baby's back. It happens. Ask me how I know.

Save money on newborn clothes by shopping consignment. It turns out you're not the only one who can't resist tiny clothes. Countless parents overshop for those first days, and their babies don't end up wearing half the stuff before they outgrow little sizes. Check out your local consignment shop. I bet you'll find a few baby outfits with the tags still on them.

If you're having a home birth, find a reason anyway to pull together a special tiny outfit. Whether it's the first outfit your parents will see them in or something to wear for their first photo shoot, allow yourself to indulge in something that can become a tiny treasure in their memory box someday.

ADULT THINGS YOU SHOULD DO,

NOW THAT YOU'RE GOING TO BE RESPONSIBLE FOR KEEPING ANOTHER HUMAN ALIVE

The list is short but each item is pretty crucial. You can do more research on why, but here's a shortlist to get you going.

- Choose a guardian for your baby in case something happens to you.

- Create a legal will so you can legally appoint that guardian.

- Learn infant CPR.

- Start a savings account for your baby.

- Take out life insurance policies for your baby, yourself, and your partner.

It's also important that you make your and your partner's health care and self-care a priority. Your baby needs healthy parents! Take advantage of maternity and paternity leave by scheduling physicals, dental visits, and eye appointments. It's common for vision to change during pregnancy, so get in ASAP in case you need to adjust your prescription.

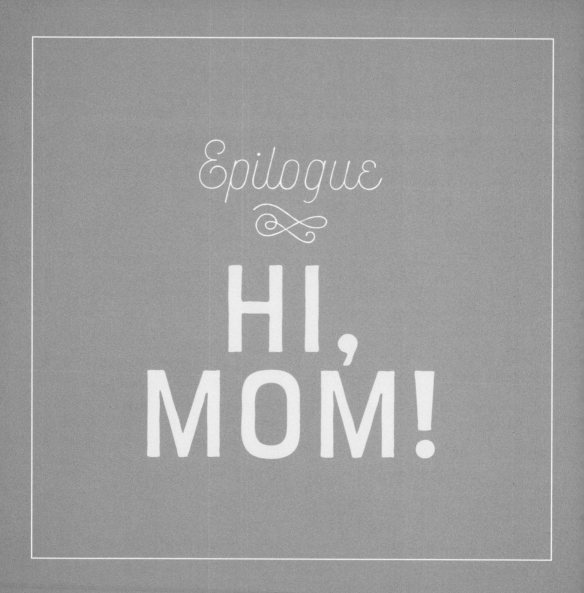

Epilogue

HI,
MOM!

*C*an you believe you just did that?! Major feels right now. I genuinely have goose bumps typing this. *Welcome to motherhood!* No matter how you got here, no matter how your baby came out of you, you have done a beautiful job! Whether you're reading this with your baby bundle snuggled on your chest because you're so obsessed with them, or you've taken a much-needed break and are locking yourself away in silence while someone else is on cuddle duty, I have no doubt you're slaying motherhood already.

I want to acknowledge that this time, what many refer to as the "fourth trimester" can be, at times, less than magical. So if you don't feel like you're doing a beautiful job, and if all this seems, well, not instinctual, please know you are not broken. You are normal. Those feelings are completely normal. The fourth trimester is all about adjusting to your new reality, so give yourself time and space and grace.

Most people think the only person experiencing transition during this time is baby. They aren't entirely wrong. Babies do have to get used to life outside of the womb. But I think mothers go through a bigger transition. You have to get used to life as a parent, your fluctuating hormones, your lactating breasts (whether or not you chose to breastfeed), and your deflating body. You're wearing mesh panties and padsicles, for goodness' sake. This is a time to be gentle on yourself and lower your expectations to ground level.

If you didn't get around to accomplishing everything on your to-do list before you went into labor, resist the urge to panic and hate yourself for it. Babies need very little to live and thrive, and you likely have access to Amazon Prime and the Internet on your phone. You can take care of your immediate needs for now and worry about the rest later. I'm going to bet that some of those things you never finished will fall off your list of priorities anyway. Babies tend to rearrange our lives like that.

But also, please give yourself a high five and some recognition for all you did get done. Whatever you managed to prepare in advance will go a long way in helping you now, and you deserve to rest.

Embrace slow days, messy bedrooms, dirty dishes, and piles of laundry. Now is not the time to try to prove to yourself or anyone else that you can balance it all. And if any of those things are really driving you nuts, don't be afraid to answer "yes" when someone reaches out and asks if there's anything they can do to help you. Visitors can do dishes, in-laws can do laundry. The most important job you can do is bond with your baby and not lose sight of your own well-being at the same time.

Three things you can do now to take care of yourself:

1. **MAKE SHOWERS OR BATHS A PRIORITY.** Hot water can feel like a heavenly trip to the spa right now. There's no reason why you should be putting off showers or baths for days at a time. Hand baby off to your partner, move the bassinet to the bathroom, or make a soft bed for baby on the floor of your bathroom and try to time your shower with a nap. The sound of the water will probably be soothing for them. And if they wake and fuss for a few minutes, it's fine. You're right there. Wash the shampoo out of your hair first before you step out.

2. **HAVE A BUFFET IN BED.** Gather all those delicious one-handed snacks you stocked, or order your favorite takeout and bring it to bed

with you. Fill your water bottle, turn on a binge-worthy show, turn off your phone, and get comfortable. Plan to spend the afternoon in bed doing nothing but relaxing and tending to your baby when they aren't napping. No visitors, no phone calls, no pants.

3. **MAKE A DATE WITH A GOOD FRIEND.** Pick a date a few weeks out when you think you'll be up to at least brushing your teeth and putting on a bra and pants, and plan to meet up with a good friend for coffee or lunch. You can plan to bring your baby or leave them with your partner (and a bottle of milk) for a bit. Either way, you'll have something to look forward to, and a reason to get out of the house.

Finally, I encourage you to go back and re-read what postpartum mental health disorder symptoms to be on the lookout for. And if you think any of those apply to you now or anytime in the next year, please reach out and get help. If your medical provider asks you questions about how you're feeling mentally at your six week postpartum checkup, answer them truthfully. It's not a pass/fail test, and there's nothing to be ashamed of. Remember that postpartum mental health disorders are treatable.

Congratulations on making it to the other side of pregnancy! I hope the last ten-ish months have instilled in you that you can do hard things, and that you have everything you need to be an awesome, imperfect, loving, real mom. I can't say the hardest parts are behind you, but I can say with certainty that the best is ahead of you.

FAQS FOR DADS-TO-BE AND NEW DADS

BY CHARLIE CAPEN, HUMORIST AND FATHER OF TWO

What do you do when you find out you're pregnant?

Have a baby. Just kidding. Your partner probably will do that. Maybe. You literally just need to learn to assist in that process and do what you can to be the best version of yourself in the coming years. Parenthood is a major commitment to a tiny human, but also to yourself. You learn things about yourself that you never could've understood without a little person depending on you. Enjoy that journey and the lessons that come with it wherever you can.

Is it normal to feel nervous, frustrated, or sad at times?

Sure. You're alive. These things can often be part of any human experience. I like to say that if you don't feel a sense of soul-crushing, existential fear, you might not be doing it right. Wondering if you're doing a good job is an indication that you care. Every emotion is on the docket when you're a dad, including some feelings of disconnectedness. Some dads don't feel a connection right away. All valid feelings.

What do I do about the controversial topics in parenthood?

I won't mention the kids here because they're all listening to every word we say. But there are some controversial parenting topics, and people have VERY intense opinions about them. As with anything involving kids, I recommend you research things thoughtfully, plan carefully, and then be willing to throw everything out the window because it's just not that easy. I was certain about where I stood on a number of parenting issues before I had kids. But that was then, and this is now. Remember that.

What kind of dad should I be?

I have no idea. Don't ask me. Ask yourself. Seriously, you can define yourself as a parent. Every time I find myself acting like some caricature of a dad (stoic dad, aggro dad, etc.), I'm not being myself. But it's up to you to figure out how to bring the best of who you are to the job at hand. The more YOU that you can be, the more you bring to your children.

Do you treat boys and girls differently?

The core process of parenting is parenting the child in front of you. They will lead you to the style of parenting they need. Do girls have to wear pink and boys wear blue? No. We only do that because we are conditioned to treat people that way. Girls do not need to be princesses by default. They could be engineers who build the castles for princesses and then take over the land ownership through their own real estate business. Why limit our kids' expression and narrow their future? You might be surprised how much we can learn from their interests and hobbies if we just let them have agency over those choices.

RESOURCES FOR NEW PARENTS

I have spent the last 10 years connecting with other parents online, and many of them have created incredible online parenting resources. I could fill an entire book with every one of them and why I love each so much, but my space here is limited. So here are a few of my favorite blogs and websites, apps, and in-person groups for moms and dads.

Blogs and Websites

BABYGUYGEARGUIDE.COM
Founder Jamie Grayson is known on Facebook and elsewhere as The Baby Guy NYC. He's an industry force, a brilliant baby gear expert, and a hilarious friend.

BABYLIST.COM
This modern solution to online baby registries lets you bring all your registries together, and it lets you add unconventional items to it, like home-cooked meals and cash for diapers or college funds.

BABYRABIES.COM
My own blog, where I share my own story and stories of other moms or would-be moms, from those trying to conceive through those parenting preschoolers.

CLICKINMOMS.COM
When you're ready to take your photography to the next level, this forum is totally worth the membership fee based on the free tutorials alone.

CLICKITUPANOTCH.COM
A great place to start if you want to improve your photography skills

COOLMOMPICKS.COM
For trusted reviews of products, apps, and services.

MAMASOFTHENICU.ORG
A community where NICU moms can come together for comfort, knowledge, and understanding. Run by a NICU mom.

MOMMYSHORTS.COM
For all things parenting and humor.

POSTPARTUM PROGRESS
The most important blog post I've ever read in my life—"The Symptoms of Postpartum Depression & Anxiety (in Plain Mama English)"—is from this site. It saved me from my own postpartum anxiety and OCD hell.

POSTPARTUM.NET
Postpartum Support International can connect any mom or anyone who cares about a mom struggling with a perinatal mood or anxiety disorder with someone who can help them.

PREGNANTCHICKEN.COM
For funny and real pregnancy talk and advice.

PROJECTNURSERY.COM
For all of your baby decor and nursery inspiration needs.

WEELICIOUS.COM
Baby, kid, and family food recipes that are simple and delicious.

WEESPRING.COM
A social shopping platform that lets you see reviews of baby gear by your friends and share your reviews with others.

Apps

WEESCHOOL

This app explains what milestones you can expect your baby to reach and when, and provides age-appropriate activities and music to play with them.

THE WONDER WEEKS

This is based on the book *The Wonder Weeks* and is a simple breakdown of the mental leaps your baby makes. It gives you an easy-to-read chart that shows exactly what leap your baby is going through and why they may be fussy.

In-Person Groups

It can feel scary to step out into the world with your baby on your own, and you might feel like just staying in would be easier. Don't do this. I say: Get out, make friends, be social. You deserve to get out there and enjoy life with your baby. Sometimes it helps to have a reason to leave the house where you know you'll be surrounded by other new parents, so here are a few groups to look into:

BARRE3.COM

There are a lot of "mommy and me" yoga classes, but what I love about Barre3 classes is that they offer child-care for babies as young as six weeks old in their small studio space, so you can really focus on yourself and also peek out the door and see that your baby is being taken care of.

BUMPCLUBANDBEYOND.COM

Based in Chicago, this social event company hosts events for moms and moms-to-be around the United States.

CITYDADSGROUP.COM

A national organization dedicated to helping fathers socialize and support one another.

MOM.ME/CLUB

A social event company hosting events in the LA area.

LIFEWITHABABY.COM

This social event company has been popular in Canada and focuses on providing emotional peer-based support. It's launching in the United States in 2018.

MOMMYCON.COM AND DADDYCON.COM

A nationwide convention series dedicated to creating and nurturing a community of parents and parents-to-be in celebration of natural parenting.

INDEX

Birthing From Within, 72

Bladder pressure, 216

Bleeding, 85–86

Bottles, 199

Bottle-sterilizing systems, 200

Bradley Method, 72

Bras, 99

Breast pads, 198

Breastfeeding

    first aid, 201

    planning for, 193–195

    pumping, 111, 208–209

    supplies, 198–199

Breathing trouble, 216–217

C

Calendula, 107

Car births, 138

Carriers, 42

Cash-back programs, 63

Cat Cow (yoga pose), 86

Certified midwives (CMs), 8–9

Certified nurse midwives
  (CNMs), 8–9

Cloth diapers, 42–44

Clothes

    baby, 105, 219–220

    bikinis, 162–163

    maternity photo shoots, 142–143

    to pack, 168–170

    shopping for maternity, 96–99

    transition pieces, 26–27

    undergarments, 99

Contraction-timing apps, 19–20

Co-sleepers, 41–42

Cravings, 58–60

Cribs, 41–42

D

Dads, 227–228

Depression, 203–206

Diaper bags, 170

Diaper covers, 43

Diaper services, 43–44

Diapers, 42–44, 62–63, 105

Diaries, 48

Digital storage, 78

DockATot, 106

Doulas, 74

Downtime, 156–157

ACKNOWLEDGMENTS

Thank you to Scott, my unwavering partner in life and parenthood, for always showing your love by supporting my whims, leaps of faith, and late nights blogging, and for rocking fatherhood in all the ways that make me feel like I won the co-parenting lottery. And for letting me sleep late most mornings.

Thank you to Kendall, Leyna, Lowell, and Wallace, my four beautifully spirited children, for pushing my buttons, opening my heart, and molding me into a better person each day. I am honestly grateful that none of you will ever let me believe I am the perfect parent I once thought I'd become. What a boring life that would be. Thank you for showing me how to embrace our wild, loud, imperfect love.

Thank you to my mom for giving me the best example of a loving mother to live up to, and to my dad for the sense of humor that has seen me through motherhood.

Thank you to Katherine Stone for writing the words that would one day show me the way out of the depths of postpartum anxiety and OCD.

Thank you to my blog readers and social media followers and friends for the support that has fueled my creativity and drive, and for the commiseration and online companionship.

Thank you to every person who helped me put this book together, from the team at Callisto Media—most especially Stacy Wagner-Kinnear and Katy Brown—to each of the book's many contributors.

ABOUT THE AUTHOR

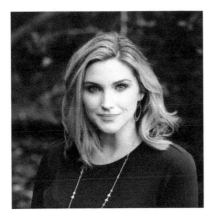

Jill Krause, née Williams, is the founder of *Baby Rabies*, an award-winning blog about pregnancy and parenthood. In the summer of 2007, Jill diagnosed herself with baby rabies—an obsession with getting pregnant, not an actual disease, y'all—and the website was born soon after (followed, appropriately, by her first child). The blog has since been recognized by a variety of media, including *TIME*, *Vogue*, *Buzzfeed*, and *The Bump*, and was awarded the 2016 Iris Award for Blog of the Year. Jill's posts and videos have been published online by outlets such as *Daily Mail*, *Us Weekly*, *Huffington Post*, *Today*, and more.

→

Jill earned her undergraduate degree in journalism from the University of Missouri, where she met her husband Scott. Together, they have four children: Kendall, Leyna, Lowell, and Wallace. In 2017, they sold their Dallas-area home and bought an RV. They are touring the country with their children the rest of 2018 and sharing that adventure on *Happy Loud Life*.

BabyRabies.com

FACEBOOK
facebook.com/BabyRabiesBlog

INSTAGRAM
BabyRabies

HappyLoudLife.com

FACEBOOK
facebook.com/HappyLoudLife

INSTAGRAM
Happy.Loud.Life

YOUTUBE
subscribe to Baby League